Anxiety

The Best TEACHER You Never Asked For

How to Turn Panic, Overthinking and Sensitivity Into Your Superpower

Sammy Barnett
Clinical Nutritionist

First published by Ultimate World Publishing 2025
Copyright © 2025 Sammy Barnett

ISBN

Paperback: 978-1-923425-61-3
Ebook: 978-1-923425-62-0

Sammy Barnett has asserted her rights under the Copyright, Designs and Patents Act 1988 to be identified as the author of this work. The information in this book is based on the author's experiences and opinions. The publisher specifically disclaims responsibility for any adverse consequences which may result from use of the information contained herein. Permission to use information has been sought by the author. Any breaches will be rectified in further editions of the book.

All rights reserved. No part of this publication may be reproduced, stored in or introduced into a retrieval system, or transmitted in any form, or by any means (electronic, mechanical, photocopying, recording or otherwise) without the prior written permission of the author. Any person who does any unauthorised act in relation to this publication may be liable to criminal prosecution and civil claims for damages. Enquiries should be made through the publisher.

Cover design: Ultimate World Publishing
Cover photo: Sumico Photography
Layout and typesetting: Ultimate World Publishing
Editor: Alex Floyd-Douglass

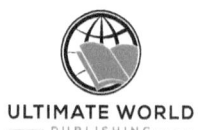

Ultimate World Publishing
Diamond Creek,
Victoria Australia 3089
www.writeabook.com.au

Nice Things People Said

"Sammy has produced a 'friend' for anxiety sufferers in her book. Not only does it clearly explain the reasons why people might find themselves on the slippery slope of anxiety and the means to overcome it, but she also elicits in the reader a greater compassion for self in the face of this challenge."

Bev Aisbett,
Counsellor, Author, Illustrator and
Artist of Anxiety

"Sammy has a gift for turning science into stories and workshops into moments of transformation. I've seen her connect with kids in ways that are both meaningful and lasting. I'm thrilled to see her bring that same energy and heart into this book. It's honest, insightful, and packed with the kind of wisdom we all wish we had growing up."

Bec Idiens,
Founder of *Lemonade Kids*, Youth Coach

"As a martial arts instructor for more than 30 years, I've seen firsthand how inner strength affects everything - from how we stand, to how we respond to challenges. Sammy's book is a powerful companion to that philosophy. She brings heart, honesty and the tools to turn anxiety into courage. It's like a black belt for the nervous system."

Master Sifu Frank Mechler,
Founder of *Freestyle Kung Fu Academy*

"Raw, real, honest, and insightful. Sammy brings a fresh and approachable look at the messy AF journey through anxiety with the perfect balance of proven research, personal experience and the Energizer Bunny quirk only she can sustain."

Jayden Leigh,
Emotions and Mindset Mastery Coach

"This book is more than a read – it's a lifeline. I've seen the pain Sammy's been through, and I've also seen her rise, time and time again. Her journey is real, raw and beautifully human. If you've ever felt like you're the only one struggling - this book will remind you that you're not."

Kassandra Kros,
Lifelong Friend

Dedication

For Liam and Tyler,

May these words be a guide when life feels heavy. I hope you find the strength to turn hard moments into lessons, fear into wisdom and anxiety into your greatest teacher.

With all my love,
Mum

Disclaimer

This book is for **informational purposes only**. While I am a qualified nutritionist, I'm not a doctor or psychologist and this isn't medical advice. Everything here is based on my experience, research and professional knowledge. It's not a substitute for professional care.

Please check in with a healthcare professional before making changes to your diet, lifestyle, or mental wellbeing.

What works for me may not work for you, so listen to your body and trust yourself. Take what helps, leave what doesn't and always seek expert advice when needed.

This book is here to guide and support you, but not to replace your doctor.

Contents

Nice Things People Said	iii
Dedication	v
Disclaimer	vii
Introduction	1
Chapter One: Born a Worrier, Not Yet a Warrior	3
Chapter Two: The Quiet Observer	17
Chapter Three: Panic at The Disco	33
Chapter Four: The Fortress of Safety	47
Chapter Five: Diagnosis: a Map or a Trap?	63
Chapter Six: Chasing Validation	83
Chapter Seven: Fighting the 'Monster'	99
Chapter Eight: The Shape Shifter	115
Chapter Nine: An A-type Awakening	137
Chapter Ten: Eating My Way to Immortality	159
Chapter Eleven: The Day My Body Quit	177
Chapter Twelve: The Woo-Woo Awakening	197
Chapter Thirteen: Learning to Sit Before We Fly	217
Chapter Fourteen: Gifts of the Sensitive Soul	235
The Afterfeels	247
About the Author	249
Gratitude Roll Call	251
The 'Nerd' Corner	253
Hungry for More?	257

Introduction

If you're holding this book, chances are you've wrestled with anxiety, overthinking, or that delightful internal monologue that won't shut up.

Welcome. I know the feeling.

I've lived it, breathed it and at times, allowed it to run my life. But here's the thing: anxiety turned out to be the best teacher I never asked for.

For years, I fought anxiety like a horror movie villain. But what if it wasn't the enemy? What if, instead of running from it, we could learn from it?

This book isn't just a collection of stories – it's a walk through my life, from my highly sensitive, slightly dramatic childhood to now. Along the way, I learnt anxiety isn't just something to survive or manage – it can guide us exactly where we're meant to be, if we let it.

I won't promise a magical fix, but I will show you a different way to see anxiety – one that might just change everything.

This book will take you on a journey of deep thoughts and even deeper feelings. My hope is that you'll laugh, feel a little seen, maybe ugly cry once or twice, and come out the other side with more clarity than you started with. Because that's life with anxiety – equal parts chaos, comedy and clarity.

So, let's get into it.

CHAPTER ONE

Born a Worrier, Not Yet a Warrior

"My first breath was followed immediately by my first worry. Was I doing it right?" (Sammy Barnett)

Even before I took my first breath, my body carried a silent tension – like it already knew the world was a lot. Sounds heavy, right? The world felt too big, too loud.

Ever clung to a parent's leg at social events? Or maybe your kids did this or still do? I once unknowingly clung to a stranger's leg at an event. Yes, I'm still recovering.

I didn't realise it, but anxiety was trying to teach me something.

Society has labelled anxiety as fear or worry – but I would soon learn it could be something else entirely. A signal. A clue. A quiet tug toward something I hadn't yet understood.

What I was learning as I clung to my mother's leg… There's safety in connection.

I wasn't weak for needing security – I was wired for it. What I didn't know yet was how to find that safety within myself.

I was the kid who sat back and watched, unsure of how to jump into the chaos that surrounded me. This feeling didn't start here though, it started well before I even took that first big breath.

Anxious in the Womb: My First Survival Training

Before I get into the science of it, let's rewind to where my story really begins – my mum's long, determined road to having me.

She tried, but it didn't always work out. My sister needed a friend, but I took over two years to arrive. At one point, I was to be Michael – until I wasn't. Eventually, she fell pregnant again and this time, it was me!

It wasn't an easy pregnancy. My mum had a threatened miscarriage the entire time and yet, I fought through. Doctors found a large tear in the placenta – I was lucky to be alive. A fighter before I even knew what I was fighting for. My sister hit the sibling jackpot. She may not have realised it at the time, but the evidence speaks for itself.

Before I was even born, I was already absorbing my mother's stress hormones. Cortisol flowing through her into me. A little stress? No big deal – our bodies are built to handle it. But chronic stress? That's like leaving the tap running. Over time, the baby's nervous system may start prepping for a world that feels intense before they're even born.

If stress hormones are pouring into the bloodstream, they may influence the baby's nervous system development. But the story doesn't stop there – postnatal bonding, environment and genetics all shape how a child experiences stress in the long run.

And the star of this stress-fuelled show? Cortisol.

NEW AND IMPROVED
TIGER JUICE

(Scientifically known as... Cortisol. But that's not nearly as fun.)

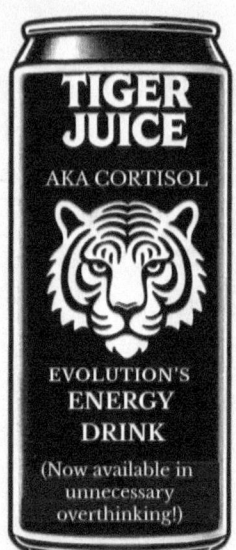

What is Tiger Juice?

The original energy shot! Brewed in your adrenal glands, sent straight to your blood.

Designed by evolution for many purposes, including:

SURVIVAL
When real tigers were lurking, Tiger Juice kicked in to:

- ☑ Spike your heart rate (**Run!**)
- ☑ Sharpen your focus (**Spot the threat!**)
- ☑ Flood your muscles with energy (**Fight, Fright, Flight, or Freeze!**)

THE PROBLEM NOW? No tigers.

Just work deadlines, phone notifications and John from accounting.

MODERN-DAY SIDE EFFECTS INCLUDE:
- ☑ Anxiety overload (Why am I spiralling over a 'K' text with NO emojis?)
- ☑ Sleep disruption (2am? Perfect time to relive that convo from 2009!)
- ☑ Digestive chaos (Pfft. Who needs digestion right?)
- ☑ Burnout (Tiger Juice: Helping you run from nothing since forever!)

HOW DO YOU TURN OFF THE TAP?
You can reset your nervous system with:
- ☑ Deep belly breathing (Your body's off-switch)
- ☑ Calm environments (No, doom-scrolling doesn't count)
- ☑ Laughter (Because if you're giggling, your body assumes the tiger left!)

THE BOTTOM LINE?

Tiger Juice was created to save you from predators, not passive-aggressive emails from John.

If you're reading this thinking, *'Great. I've doomed my baby.'* Breathe. Stress can be passed down – but so can calm. That's our power.

I carried guilt for years after learning this, replaying every stressful moment from my pregnancies. But here's what I wish I had known sooner.

Our nervous systems aren't stuck. **They adapt.**

Babies aren't born with a life sentence of anxiety – they're born with a nervous system that responds to its environment. And the good news? We can change that environment, even after birth.

Stress signals tell the baby the world is tough. But calm, connection? They say, *'You are safe. You are okay.'*

And that message? It rewires everything.

What if, when we were pregnant, we did simple things? Belly breathing. Soft music. Laughing with friends.

What if we let our bodies send a message to the baby that the world isn't always a threat? That it's okay out here. That we don't have to be on high alert all the time.

The Unwanted Family Heirloom

The thing is, sometimes we do everything 'right' and our babies still come out feeling anxious. Trauma doesn't just live in our experiences – it can be passed down.

Studies on the children and grandchildren of Holocaust survivors reveal they were born with distinct stress hormone profiles. They often showed altered cortisol regulation, even though they never lived through war themselves. Their little bodies were pre-programmed to expect stress. Trauma doesn't just leave scars – it rewires how future generations respond to the world.

Research found that children of Holocaust survivors with PTSD have lower cortisol levels (Yehuda & Lehrner, 2018), not higher. And just to clear cortisol's name here – it's not all that bad. In healthy amounts, it's essential. It helps regulate our energy and reduce inflammation. It's nature's in-built recovery system – but when it's out of whack, everything else follows.

If someone has consistently low baseline cortisol, it may mean their system is worn out or dysregulated. Meaning these children were wired to expect stress, their body always scanning for threats because it didn't trust it would recover easily.

Even at the genetic level, trauma leaves its mark. Studies show it can tweak the very genes that regulate stress, passing down a blueprint like an unwanted family heirloom (Yehuda et. Al, 2016).

Trauma? Could it be the ultimate family heirloom?

But here's the twist. Maybe some of us were built for this. Maybe anxiety is a superpower.

In ancient tribes, who do you think spotted the tigers first? The anxious ones. Maybe we aren't weak – maybe we are the original security system. Our nervous system isn't broken. It's running outdated software in a world that doesn't need that much surveillance anymore.

Anxiety is passing down survival strategies like an old family recipe. It's saying, *'Be ready. Stay aware.'*

The problem? The threats have changed and no one has given it time to rewrite the program.

Good news. Just because our parents or grandparents lived through trauma, doesn't mean we have to carry it forward. We can rewrite the blueprint for our children.

Healing, too, can be inherited.

But I hadn't figured that out, I was just a kid – wired for survival, but with no tigers in sight. Just everyday life, which, to my nervous system, was apparently just as terrifying.

The First Signs of Panic

So here I was, in the world, anxious about everything, not knowing why. How do I know I was feeling this way? Because I've heard the stories – from family and friends. I was the quiet, shy child. The weird, sensitive, deeply attached-to-my-mother child.

What's your first memory of feeling anxious? First day at school? A sleepover gone wrong? Or that time *Toy Story* made you side-eye your stuffed animals at night. No? Just me?

I'm sure many of you have seen children like this. Maybe you have a child like this and that's okay. As you keep reading, you'll see that being wired this way isn't a curse – it's a gift. You just need to know how to use it.

My mum was my anchor. My safety. The world was fast, loud and overwhelming. What I didn't know was that my mum was feeling everything I was feeling, too. I was her anchor just as much as she was mine. We were tethered to each other.

We did everything together. Family outings. Movie matinees. My mum has fond memories of taking me to see *Pretty Woman*. Meanwhile, I had no idea what a prostitute was – just that Julia Roberts got a really nice makeover.

At family gatherings, I was the quiet observer. My sister did the talking for me. I needed my mum in the same room – my safety net, my anchor. As long as she was there, I could handle the noise, the people, the chaos.

But then along came kindergarten. One day a week, a gentle introduction to school. Except to me, it wasn't gentle – it was a tether being cut.

The drive there? Pure terror. My little body knew what was coming. I clung to my mum like my life depended on it – because to my nervous system, it did. I fought like a cornered animal. Kicked. Bit. Screamed. This wasn't just 'separation anxiety' – this was my whole world being ripped away.

'Do not leave me in this unsafe place!'

Anxiety was screaming at me, *'This is unfamiliar! Stay close to safety!'*

But what it didn't know? I had to learn, step by step, that I could handle new experiences. My nervous system wasn't broken – it was just running outdated software.

I see this all the time in anxious children. I saw it in my youngest. He was the one I kept home the longest, the one I anchored into when I felt anxious. We fed off each other.

And when I run my kids' workshops, I hear the same thing from parents. *'My child is extremely anxious. They don't want to leave me. They won't go to school.'*

Then I talk to the parent and I see it – the same anxious feelings. I can sense it.

Children are like little emotional sponges – they soak up everything, from our words to our worries and actions. But it's not just about 'catching' anxiety. Genetics, personality and life experiences all play a role in shaping how they move through the world.

So, if your kid avoids phone calls, dodges conflict and needs a cooling-off period before answering texts – yeah, they might be mirroring you.

It's a cycle. I sometimes hold up the proverbial mirror and see parents breakdown – because deep down, they already know.

Now, I'm not saying abandon your child. I am saying that sometimes, as anxious parents, we anchor into our children instead of understanding anxiety within ourselves. In neglecting our own feelings, we teach them to do the same – teaching the same lessons.

Parenting: The Team Sport That We Somehow Made a Solo Mission

Once upon a time, children weren't raised in isolation. Parenting wasn't a one-person (or two-person) job – it was a tribal effort. Babies were passed around, kids played in groups and multiple caregivers shared the emotional load. A stressed-out parent wasn't left to figure it all out alone – they had aunties, elders and a village to help regulate not just the baby, but themselves.

Now? Many parents are trying to do it all – work, cook, clean, emotionally support their kids and somehow stay sane – alone. No wonder so many of us are running on stress fumes. Our nervous systems are wired for support, for shared responsibility.

Instead, in the Western world, we've swapped the village for overstimulation, 24/7 work demands and constant pressure to get it right. Children pick up on this stress, not because parents are failing, but because the system wasn't designed for this.

If you're feeling overwhelmed as a parent, you're not alone. Parenting was never designed to be a solo gig. Support can make all the difference.

Our nervous systems weren't just wired to run from tigers – they were also designed to keep us connected. Back in ancient times, being alone or outcast wasn't just lonely, it was dangerous. Survival depended on the tribe. From a young age, we seek connection for safety. When that safe person leaves – whether it's a parent stepping out or a child being left at school – the alarm bells ring. It doesn't distinguish between a real threat and an imagined one. It just knows that, historically, being alone could mean danger.

I've learnt that stepping back – not neglecting, not ignoring, but not feeding the anxiety 'monster' – helped my child thrive. Because here's the thing: anxiety isn't a monster at all. It's a feeling – one that's often misunderstood. But once he understood it, once he tapped into it, it started to become a powerful tool. This is one we don't want our children to fear, but to learn from.

As the years went on, that anxious feeling never left me. For some children, anxiety shows up in small ways – fear of swimming, riding a bike. For me, it was everywhere. My mind absorbed everything – especially fear. Even movies weren't just entertainment, they were fuel for my imagination. They turned everyday worries into full-blown terrors.

Anxiety: The Best TEACHER You Never Asked For

THE ANXIOUS BRAIN THEATRE

(Where overactive imaginations run wild!)

Produced by my brain – starring me.

Act 1.
BELLYBUTTON DROP-OFF

I overheard a mum say her baby's bellybutton was about to fall off. Wait... Is that a thing?! Cue checking my bellybutton hourly like it's on a countdown timer.

Act 2.
FORGETTING TO BREATHE

What if I just forgot how? Or my body suddenly went on strike? I spent nights manually breathing, terrified I'd miss a breath.

Act 3.
BATHTUB VORTEX OF DOOM

Do NOT unplug the bath while I'm still in here! I will be sucked down the pipes and end up who-knows-where.

Act 4.
SWALLOWING A SEED

The day I ate a watermelon seed was the day I accepted my fate: Vines would soon sprout from my ears and I'd become half-human, half-fruit.

What ridiculous fears has your anxious brain cooked up?

Anxiety was always scanning, always on high alert. But it couldn't tell the difference between real danger from my overactive imagination. It was just trying to keep me safe – even if that meant preparing for threats that didn't exist.

Little did I know, this was just the beginning. Anxiety wasn't the villain of my story – it was the teacher. And I? The reluctant student sitting in the back, questioning everything.

ANXIETY CHEAT SHEET: What You Need to Know

The way we regulate our own nervous system can shape the next generation.

Lesson 1: Anxiety Runs in Families, But So Does Healing
If a child is anxious, it doesn't mean you've failed – it could mean you're an important source of support for them.

TRY THIS: When a child is anxious, start with yourself. Take a deep breath, plant your feet and reset – your calm is contagious. But if regulating feels impossible – because, let's be real, some days it is – know that support is out there. Therapy, tools, your community – whatever helps. Every situation is different and you don't have to do it alone.

Lesson 2: We Weren't Meant to Raise Children Alone
Humans are wired for community. Parenting was never meant to be a one-person (or even two-person) job. Support systems matter – for you and your child.

TRY THIS: Build your village. If you feel overwhelmed, ask yourself: *Who or what helps me feel supported?* Anxiety thrives in isolation – but connection, whether through family, friends, or professionals, can help.

REMINDER: Your child doesn't need a 'perfect' parent. They just need a safe one.

CHAPTER TWO

The Quiet Observer

*"Do not underestimate the silent ones.
They watch, they learn and they grow."* (Unknown)

While chaos swirled around me, I found safety in silence. When you're the quiet one, others tend to speak for you.

My cousin, just four weeks older, often took the lead – bold, opinionated, unafraid. I envied her ability to own a room but resented how easily her voice became my voice.

She spoke. People listened. My words? Trapped behind an invisible wall like they were something to be ashamed of.

I wasn't sure what stung more – being unheard or knowing I kept myself silent.

I could've gone through childhood without speaking. If there was a 'Spokesperson of the Year' award, my cousin would've won every time. I was just the silent sidekick, nodding along like a human emoji.

My sister spoke for me.

My mum spoke for me.

There was rarely a need for me to use my own voice.

But don't worry, I'm making up for lost time – now I get paid to speak. I've got a lot to say. Just ask my husband.

When Silence Feels Safe

At school, I spoke even less. The fear of saying the wrong thing was paralysing.

What if they laughed at me? What if I liked something no one else did? Better to blend in. Primal instincts.

Turns out, anxiety thought it was protecting me from social 'death'. It's logic.

If you don't speak, you can't say something silly.

If you don't say something silly, you won't get rejected.

If you don't get rejected, you'll be safe.

Airtight, right? Except that's not how life works. I learnt this the hard way.

One day, my teacher falsely accused a classmate. Before I could stop myself, I blurted, *'That's not what happened!'*

The class stared. My heart pounded.

The teacher snapped, *'Be quiet, Samantha!'*

The shame burned. I replayed it in my mind for weeks. Anxiety made sure I paid the price: *'See? This is why we don't speak up.'*

So, I didn't. Not for a long time.

Anxiety thought it was doing me a favour – keeping me safe from embarrassment, rejection and being wrong. But it wasn't just silencing me. It was training me.

For people with social anxiety, the amygdala – the brain's fear centre – overreacts, treating small things like life-or-death. Of course, anxiety isn't just one part of the brain – it's a whole network. But the amygdala? That guy pulls the fire alarm for burnt toast.

MEET YOUR PRINCIPAL
Ms. AMY. G DALA

Your Amygdala

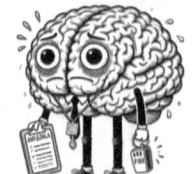

The Overprotective School Principal

What's Happening?

Your amygdala?

It's in charge of keeping you safe, whether that means getting you out of the way of an oncoming bus (actual danger) or making sure you don't say something silly in class (perceived danger).

Do They Learn?

YES!

Every time you face a fear and don't die, the amygdala and anxiety update their notes.

How Anxiety Fits:

Anxiety, the over-prepared teacher taking notes from the amygdala and then just runs with them. The amygdala overreacts, pulls the fire alarm for a burnt piece of toast. Anxiety, thinking the alarm is legit, starts prepping you for survival – cue racing heart, overthinking and panic.

Instead of fighting with the teacher, give her feedback. Prove that you're safe. The more you show up despite fear, the more your brain rewires itself to chill.

So, maybe we don't need a fire drill every time we speak up?

And if the amygdala overreacts to speaking up, you can bet it goes into full-blown meltdown when there's even a hint of rejection.

Rejection Feels Like A Punch to the Gut

Ever said *'Hi'* to someone and got nothing back? Brain meltdown initiated. That's Principal Amygdala in full panic mode. *'Welp, that's it! We had a good run. Guess we're going into witness protection now.'*

Our brains are wired for belonging, which is why rejection stings so much – it physically hurts. Studies show social rejection activates the same brain regions as actual pain (Eisenberger et al., 2003).

We're using an outdated textbook. Rejection isn't the end of the world – that anxious feeling is proof that you showed up. And showing up is how we get better at anything.

The One-Friend Safety Net

At school, I always found that *one* safe person – the friend who accepted me as I was (or at least as much of me as I allowed them to see).

It was freeing. It also made me dependent on that one friend. If they weren't there, I felt lost.

Children with more than one friend? Studies say they bounce back better (Bukowski et al., 2010). I didn't know that at the time. My best friend was my security blanket and the idea of branching out? Terrifying!

I see this in children today – the ones who cling to one friend. It's beautiful, but it can also be limiting. My son was the same. Until it became a problem. He struggled to connect outside that one friendship and when that friend was away, anxious feelings took off. No security net.

I saw myself in him.

It's okay to have one friend, but if that friendship becomes a security blanket? It can hold you back from growing.

The Yes Girl

I feared being too much or not enough, so I adapted. Blended in. Made sure I was easy to be around.

I became the 'Yes Girl' – agreeable, easy-going and always seeking approval.

'No strong opinions of your own, Samantha. It's safer to stay neutral.'

Until it's not.

Anxiety taught me that saying *'yes'* kept me safe. But in reality? Saying *'yes'* to everything meant saying *'no'* to myself.

Eventually, I had to unlearn the idea that keeping others comfortable was more important than my own needs.

But for now, the 'Yes Girl' was on her way to becoming a full pledged people-pleaser.

Ever find yourself agreeing to something and then immediately regretting it? Like, *'Sure, I'll help you move boxes this weekend!'* Then suddenly it's Saturday morning, you're rearranging your children, so you can lift boxes for a lady you just met down the road – questioning every life choice that led you here.

When Still Waters Are Seen As Shallow

I was quiet for so long that many people assumed I was lacking intelligence. The slow one. The kid who would never amount to much.

It's wild how quickly some people mistake silence for lack of intelligence.

As Susan Cain points out in *Quiet* (2012), *"Our culture is biased against quiet and reserved people, but introverts are responsible for some of humanity's greatest achievements."*

And yet, if you're not the loudest in the room, many people assume you have nothing to say.

The problem? When you hear something enough – even if it's not true – you start to believe it. Words carry weight. Labels? They're sticky. Sometimes we shrink to fit them, sometimes we fight against them. But either way, they leave a mark. Research shows just how powerful expectations can be. When someone believes in us, we tend to step up. And when they don't… Well, that can change everything too. (Rosenthal and Jacobson, 1968)

In my case? I leaned into them without even realising it. The more people assumed I had nothing to offer, the more I shrank. Even though deep down, I knew I had more to say.

So later in life, I overcompensated. I worked twice as hard, spoke twice as much and went out of my way to prove to the world (and myself) that I was not lacking intelligence.

And I would see this all the time in clinic. Women who felt small, who hesitate before sharing an idea because they don't want to sound silly. These feelings didn't appear overnight.

For generations, women have been conditioned to stay quiet, to smile and nod, to be 'nice'. And even now, in modern society, we still see brilliant women doubting their own voices.

But here's the thing:

Each time a woman speaks up – even if her voice shakes – she's disrupting that patten.

Your voice matters.

Your ideas matter.

And every time you speak up, you're not just breaking your silence – you're breaking centuries of silence.

But what if being quiet wasn't something to overcome? What if silence was your superpower – the kind that watches, listens, absorbs every detail, every shift in tone, every unspoken word?

Turns out, I wasn't just the quiet one. I was the observer.

From Quiet to Hyper-Aware

I could pick up on emotions, the tiniest shifts in tone, the things people weren't saying. Some people call this being a *'Highly Sensitive Person (HSP)'* – a term coined by psychologist

Dr. Elaine Aron to describe people who feel everything, like emotional sponges.

Sound familiar? Same.

It's a gift, but when you don't know how to manage it? It's exhausting.

I thought everyone could sense energy shifts the way I did. Spoiler: They couldn't. And because I could feel them, I thought it was my job to fix them.

- ➢ If someone had a bad day, I felt like it was my fault.
- ➢ If someone was upset, I absorbed it like a sponge.

I carried the weight of everyone else's emotions while silently drowning in my own.

Turns out, when you spend your whole life hyper-aware of every little shift in energy, you develop a freakishly accurate radar for people's emotions. Even the ones they think they're hiding.

Anxiety: The Best TEACHER You Never Asked For

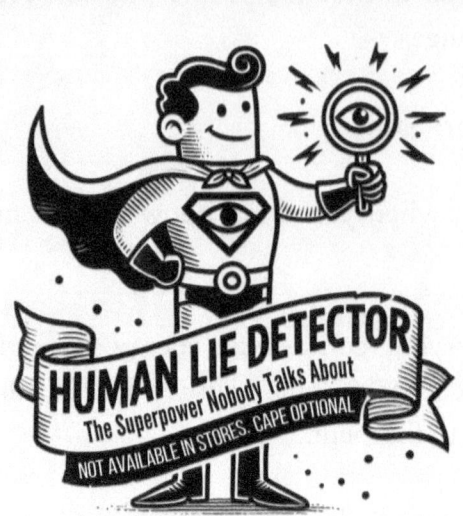

Congratulations!

If you've spent a lifetime watching, listening and reading the room like an FBI agent, you may have unlocked a rare superpower of Hyper-Awareness Mode.

The Perks of This Highly Underrated Skill:

- You know when someone's really fine vs. 'I'm fine.'
- You can sense tension in the air before anyone even speaks.
- You can detect sarcasm at extreme levels.
- You see micro-expressions people don't even know they're making.

The Downside?

- You also sense vibes that aren't yours to fix.
- You read way too much into a one-word text...with no emojis! Who does that!?
- People lie and you let them think they got away with it.

What to Do With This Superpower?

- Use it wisely. Not everyone wants their emotions analysed.
- Set boundaries. Just because you can feel someone's energy shift doesn't mean it's your job to fix it – funny that.
- Own it. If people call you too sensitive, remind them that noticing what's unspoken is a rare skill – one that makes you a secret weapon.

'I see through your nonsense, John. Proceed with caution.'

Anxiety trained me to be a human lie detector. That can be a superpower – if you use it wisely. But it can also be exhausting if you're constantly scanning for danger that isn't there.

Anxiety meant well, but sometimes it was just looking for problems that didn't exist. And when there weren't any real threats to obsess over? It found a new target – *me*.

Anxiety's Quality Control Department

My brain ran quality control on every interaction. A social blooper from 10 years ago? It remembered. A better way I could have worded something? Anxiety had notes.

Which is how I got stuck with an unpaid, overactive inner voice.

Anxiety: The Best TEACHER You Never Asked For

YOUR INNER VOICE
The Roommate Who Won't SHUT UP

If you talk to yourself more than you talk to actual humans, congrats! You're normal. Research shows the average person has more than 6,000 thoughts a day (Poppenk & Tseng, 2020) – and let's say 5,000 of them are just you arguing with yourself.

Your inner voice is like a roommate who never moved out – always critiquing, overanalysing and reminding you about that awkward thing you said back in 2008 to John. Sorry John.

Why did you wave at that person, they weren't waving at you! Idiot.

They said HOW are you? Not, WHO are you? You sounded like an Idiot.

Raise your hand if your brain has ever brought up something embarrassing from 10 years ago at 2am.

Oh good, just me? Cool, cool, cool.

The Good News?

You can train your inner roommate to stop being such a jerk, even at 2am! Your brain learns from repetition — so if you start feeding it better scripts, it eventually adapts.

TRY THIS:

Give your inner critic a ridiculous name (Petunia? Kevin? John?).
Next time they start running their mouth, respond with:

'Not today, John. We're doing the thing.'
'Kevin, I appreciate the input, but I'm speaking up anyway'.

Upgrade your self-talk like you're hyping up a friend:

'Okay, I might stumble, but that's proof I'm trying.'
'I am allowed to take up space.'
'I am more interesting than Petunia thinks.'

Why This Works

Science shows that what we tell ourselves on repeat becomes our reality. If your current inner voice sounds like a nervous apprentice, it's time to upgrade to Samuel L. Jackson mode.

Ask yourself: Would Samuel L. Jackson question whether or not he should speak up? No, he would say the thing with authority and probably throw in some very colourful language:

"Say 'what' again?! I dare you, I double dare you motherf****r!" (Pulp Fiction, 1994)

With all that noise in my head, I needed somewhere safe to put my thoughts. Somewhere they wouldn't be judged, analysed, or thrown back at me. And for a while, that place wasn't a person. It was a dog.

Confessions to a Cocker Spaniel

When I was about four or five years old, the only one I could confide in was Becky, the neighbours' cocker spaniel. Every day after school, she'd run down to me. I would tell her everything – unpacking the events of the day. Unpacking the day with someone? Essential. Even if it's a dog. It was here that I fell in love with the dog. What wonderful little furry angels that have been gifted to humans.

Who was your childhood safe space? A pet? A stuffed animal? That one adult who actually listened to you? Or were you like me, trauma-dumping on a dog? Maybe you still do? Maybe I still do?

Becky and I would lay in the backyard, staring at the sky – well, *I'd* stare at the sky while she panted and waited for belly rubs. She listened. And in those moments, everything felt right in the world.

I didn't know then how much I needed her. Or how much it would hurt when she was gone.

The Day My Safe Space Disappeared

One day, I came home from school and my mum told me Becky had gone to heaven. A twisted stomach. An operation the neighbours couldn't afford. I never saw her again. I never got to say goodbye.

Child psychologists say that losing a pet is often a child's first experience with real grief – and it can bring up big, existential questions. I was no exception. Becky wasn't just a dog; she was my safe space. Losing her cracked open a door in my mind that I couldn't close, *'What happens when we die?'*

I spiralled. My mind latched onto this new fear, *'I could die? Everyone dies at some point?'*

If you've ever been around a child afraid of death, you know how consuming it can be. I've met many children who absorb everything, feel everything and have no idea what to do with it. Children who are trapped in their own heads, just like I was.

Looking back, I see that anxiety wasn't *just* freaking out – it was trying to prepare me for the unknown. But some things in life? You can't prepare for. You must live them.

And yet, I couldn't just let it go. My brain wasn't wired that way. If there was a question, I needed an answer. And if there was no answer? I'd go searching for one.

The First Time I Asked Big Questions

I went to a Catholic school, though my family wasn't religious. Still, I was always searching for something more – something bigger. And when the questions about life and death took over my mind, I sought answers.

There was a priest at my school. People said you could talk to him about anything. So I did.

Why was I born? What happens when we die? What is the meaning of life? If God created everything, who created God?

He didn't have all the answers, but at least he listened. And maybe that was the point. Maybe the real comfort wasn't in the answers, but in knowing someone was willing to listen.

I spent so much time in my head – watching, thinking, feeling. I used to see it as a flaw, punishing myself for overanalysing everything.

And now, looking back, I see those silent years for what they were.

I wasn't just a quiet girl.

I was becoming something else entirely.

ANXIETY CHEAT SHEET:
What You Need to Know

Anxiety didn't make me quiet – it made me watch. It turned me into a human lie detector, an emotional sponge and an overthinker.

Lesson 1: Silence Isn't Always Safety
Anxiety says stay quiet to avoid messing up. But staying small isn't protection – it can become a prison.

TRY THIS: Say *one* uncomfortable thing daily. An opinion. A question. A simple *hi*. Every time you do, your brain updates its notes. Speaking doesn't equal danger.

Lesson 2: Not Every Emotion Is Yours to Fix
You may pick up on shifts, tension and the unspoken, but just because you *sense* something doesn't mean it's your job to solve it.

TRY THIS: Before assuming it's about you, pause. Ask, *'Did they actually say something, or am I filling in the blanks?'*

REMINDER: You're allowed to take up space.

CHAPTER THREE

Panic at The Disco

"Who needs roller coasters when your body randomly decides to scare you for free?"
(Sammy Barnett)

Imagine an invisible hand gripping your chest, the world spins out of control. Your body projects you into another plane. All you can think is: *'This is it. I am dying!'*

Now imagine you're 11 years old and this is happening at least 10 times a day. This wasn't just a bad moment – it was my new reality. An uninvited guest that refused to leave.

Up until this moment, I had been afraid, sure, but I had still been *doing*. I showed up at school. I hung out with friends, who made me feel safe. I was slowly becoming more resilient. I was growing into myself.

But I was still the 'Yes Girl'. I still didn't know how to express myself. Like most children at that age, I was just trying to fit in, trying to find my tribe.

We had discos, parties and sleepovers. It was all fun – laughing, dancing and feeling like life was somewhat simple. Until one night, everything changed.

The Night My World Split in Two

Let's set the scene. I was at a disco in our primary school hall. The excitement was next-level, as it always was at that age.

And then, the *Macarena* song came on.

You know the dance. You're probably singing the song in your head right now if you speak Spanish. Maybe you're humming it.

I was ready. I had the moves. Hands out, flip, flip, shoulder, shoulder, hip – *and then my soul left my body.* One second I was about to break it down and the next, my body decided it was being chased by an axe murderer.

I thought the *Macarena* was harmless – until that night. If the *Macarena* was a portal to hell, I had accidentally unlocked it.

The music pulsed through me, vibrating in my chest. Then, suddenly, it dissolved into an eerie, slowed silence in the background. I could feel my heartbeat hammering loudly in my chest all the way up into my throat, louder, louder, faster, faster. My vision shattered into a blur of dark colours and haze that made me lightheaded and dizzy. Faces and bodies swirling around me of concern and laughter. Familiar faces turning into strangers. Every muscle and nerve in my body felt like it was shutting down as a tidal wave of terror came crashing over me.

In a split second, I was no longer in my body.

The ground beneath me seemed to crumble away and the Earth begun to swallow me whole. I had no option but to float helplessly in a vast disorientating void. Desperation and panic drove me to reach out to anything that could stop me from being swallowed up or float away. Something real in this world to pull me away from the unknown abyss beneath me. My hands were cold and clammy, my stomach in knots.

'This is it. This is how I will die.'

In that fleeting moment, I experienced the most profound terror of my life – a silent, internal apocalypse that no one else could see. Yet one that left me utterly and permanently changed…forever.

I ran.

I bolted out the hall, threw myself onto the ground, trying to make the world stop spinning, trying to stop *whatever this was* from completely taking over.

I was only 11. I had no idea what had just happened to me.

Everyone was trying to help – checking if I was okay – but I couldn't explain it.

I didn't know how to.

I was shaking, my breath shallow, but the cool night air wrapped around me like a safety net. My cousin and friend followed me out, sitting down on the grass beside me, their faces with worry. I could barely process their words, but I knew they were there. That helped.

I felt the earth beneath me, solid and unmoving. My body knew what it needed – I lay back in the grass, feeling the dampness seep through my clothes, looking up at the vast, open sky. The universe felt huge – my panic small in comparison.

A teacher crouched beside me. *"It's overwhelming in there, huh?"* she said gently. *"Hot, loud…too much."*

Yes. Too much.

Eventually, the panic began to fade – not gone, but retreating, like a tide pulling back just enough for me to catch my breath. I tried going back inside, but the moment I stepped through the doors, the wave crashed over me again.

Nope. Not happening.

I stayed put outside, the cool breeze brushing over my skin, my heartbeat still unsteady but slowing. The disco kept going, laughter and music spilling into the night, but I stayed where I was, grounded in the dirt, waiting for my body to remember that I was safe.

No one really talked about panic attacks in children back then. It wasn't a common *thing*. No one knew what was 'wrong' with me.

And that was the most terrifying part. I had no answers. I was alone in this. At least, that's what it felt like.

This thing would be with me every day for years to come.

What I didn't know then was that my body wasn't actually broken – it was just wildly misinformed. It thought I was in danger and was doing everything in its power to save me. The problem? There was no danger. My brain was like a malfunctioning school fire alarm – blaring at full volume even when there was no real fire.

Which brings me to this.

EMERGENCY PROTOCOL
FALSE ALARM EDITION

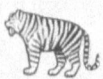

— ★ No actual danger. Your brain is just being dramatic. ★ —

ALERT STATUS: Panic Mode Activated

Trigger Detected! Your brain thinks there's a life-threatening emergency.

Reality Check! There is no actual fire. You just burnt the toast again.

Emergency Response Plan

Step 1: Principal Amygdala Sounds Alarm	Step 2: Tiger Juice Deployment	Step 3: All Systems Abandon Ship	Step 4: Full-Blown Chaos Ensues
He's freaking out over...well, nothing. He slams the panic button and sends your body into full evacuation mode. Cue theme music: **Highway to the Danger Zone** blares in the background.	Your body is flooded with Tiger Juice (a cocktail of adrenaline and cortisol). Heart races, breathing speeds up – obviously, we need to escape this invisible danger!	Logical thinking? Evacuated. Digestion? Shut down until further notice. Calmness? Nowhere to be found.	You're dizzy, nauseous and 100% convinced you're dying. Spoiler: You're not. It's just a fire drill for a fire that doesn't exist.

FALSE ALARM PROCEDURE

- Stay put: You do NOT need to run. The alarm is malfunctioning.
- Announce the glitch: Say (out loud or in your head): 'This is a false alarm. I am safe'
- Breathe Like a cool, collected firefighter: Slow, deep breaths tell your body there's no emergency.
- Wait for the all-clear: Panic can't last forever. Ride the wave and it will fade.

FINAL NOTICE: Principal Amygdala Needs a Vacation

Your brain is not broken. It's just overactive at threat detection.
With practice, you can teach it to chill –
so you don't keep evacuating over burnt toast.

For years, I thought panic was my enemy, a monster sent to ruin my life. But what if it wasn't?

What if it was just my body, desperately trying to protect me in the only way it knew how?

The more I fought it, the louder it screamed. The lesson? Sometimes, the only way to quieten the alarm is to stop running and start listening.

At this point, I had no clue what any of this meant. This was my first experience. I didn't know my amygdala was completely unhinged, nor did I realise this was just the beginning.

A long battle lay ahead – one that I had no choice but to face.

But at that moment, I didn't know any of that. All I knew was that I wanted to forget.

The Panic Aftermath

That night, I went home with my friend, still rattled but trying to push it away.

Maybe it was just a *weird* thing. Maybe it was *nothing*.

Just as I began to relax, hoping it was a one-time thing – it struck again!

I was at a friend's sleepover when the panic hit again, I had to wake her mum to call my mum – an absolutely terrifying task in itself.

I thought I was dying. Again!

Back home, I felt a little better – but I wasn't the same.

I knew, deep in my bones, something had shifted. My life had just split into two.

Before. And after.

And *after* was a terrifying place to be.

In that moment, anxiety wasn't a teacher – it was a monster, hijacking my body and taking me hostage with no ransom note. I didn't know it yet, but it wasn't just there to torment me.

It was screaming for my attention.

Not to be feared. To be understood.

I grieved the *before* version of me for years, convinced she was lost forever. What I didn't yet realise was that *after* me wasn't broken – she was being rebuilt.

At the time, anxiety felt like my enemy. But looking back, it forced me to ask questions no one else was asking:

What was my body trying to tell me?

What needed to change?

Diagnosis: Unknown

My 'mystery illness' baffled everyone.

I was called a hypochondriac. I had too many things going on in my body for it to be real. They thought I was making it up.

But I wasn't.

It was happening. At least 10 times a day. It followed me *everywhere*. It felt like a demonic force flinging open the gates of hell, dragging me into a nightmarish abyss – but no Constantine, let alone Keanu Reeves. My only heroic response was a flurry of wildly flailing arms and a sprint to the nearest exit.

I wasn't *safe*. I needed Keanu to burst through the door and save me.

My mum wanted answers. She took me to doctors – blood tests, CAT scans, specialists.

Nothing. No explanations. Just more frustration, more isolation.

If Doctor Google existed back then, I'd have diagnosed myself with everything from chronic dehydration to an undetectable rare disease. I was basically a medical mystery. Like *House*, but with 'too many feelings' instead of lupus.

I even started questioning myself.

Am I making this up?
Am I going crazy already?

No. I *felt* it. It was real. So why couldn't anyone *see* it?

For most of my childhood, I had a safe space. Life was predictable. But something shifted when I was nine. The undercurrent of pain, heartache and uncertainty seeped into our home. My parents' marriage was unravelling and even though no one said it outright, I felt the tension, the unspoken sadness lingering in the walls.

When the panic attacks started, the assumption was clear: *She's just looking for attention.*

The school counsellor became my designated support person, but no one really knew what to do with me. There was no diagnosis, no explanation – just the quiet, underlying belief that maybe, if I just *tried harder*, I could stop.

For a long time, I suffered in silence so as not to draw attention to me.

What no one knew then – including me – was that childhood stress rewires the body in ways we don't fully understand until later. When a child experiences ongoing emotional distress, unpredictability, or fear (like watching a family fall apart), the brain starts over-preparing for danger. It learns to be on edge, scanning for threats, overreacting to even minor changes.

These kinds of early life stressors don't just shape behaviour – they shape biology. Research shows they can lead to long-term inflammatory change in the body that can increase the risk for mental illness (Danese & Baldwin, 2017).

This is why panic isn't just about *'thinking too much'* or *'being dramatic'*. For many of us, it's about a nervous system that learnt to be afraid.

And that's not something you can just 'snap out of'.

The Impact of Being Misunderstood

When a child is dismissed, they don't stop feeling what they're feeling. *They just stop trusting themselves and those around them.*

Being called *'overly sensitive'* or told to *'just stop worrying'* doesn't erase the fear – it buries it deep within. It turns doubt inward, making you question yourself.

Was I making this up? Was something wrong with me?

When no one believed me, I started believing them. Maybe I was overreacting. Maybe I was broken. But looking back, I can see what I couldn't then – anxiety wasn't trying to ruin me. It was trying to tell me something. It was a signal, not a villain.

But what made it worse wasn't just the panic itself – it was how other people reacted to it.

Panic in the Public Eye

Panic doesn't stay hidden for long.

It wasn't just a *me* problem anymore. It was happening everywhere. At school. In front of people. In moments when I just wanted to be invisible.

The body stays on high alert, waiting for the next attack. Scanning. Bracing. Preparing.

Panic didn't discriminate – school parades? Nope. Open spaces? Closed spaces? Crowds? It found me everywhere.

What started privately quickly spilled into my public life, turning everyday moments into humiliating spectacles.

At school, I became *that* girl. The weird one. The one who couldn't control her body. The one people whispered about.

'Why can't she just stop it?'
'Is it happening again?'
'She's looking for attention.'

Attention?! The last thing I wanted was more eyes on me.

And then, what felt like depression crept in.

I didn't know it was depression at the time, but looking back, I see it so clearly. I felt *different*. *Wrong*. Like everyone else had a map and I was lost in a place I didn't belong.

My only comfort was my tiny, Chihuahua-Maltese fluffball. She didn't care that I was basically a walking disaster. She just curled up beside me, no questions asked. I felt like she had more emotional intelligence than most adults.

But nothing else helped. The questions in my head never stopped.

Why was my body doing this?

Why was it betraying me?

Why couldn't I just be normal?

Shame. Embarrassment. Self-loathing. The perfect recipe to feed the fear.

So, I found the only solution that made sense. Avoid everything.

If I didn't go, I wouldn't panic. If I just stayed home, I wouldn't have to deal with the fear.

It felt safe. But here's the cruel trick: Avoidance teaches your brain that the world is more dangerous than it actually is.

Every time I skipped something, my brain said, '*See? You survived because you stayed away.*'

I didn't know it yet, but this decision would shape years of my life.

It would change how I saw the world. How I saw myself.

And worst of all? It would make panic even more powerful.

That was the lesson – fear grows when you run from it. The only way to shrink it is to turn around and face it.

ANXIETY CHEAT SHEET: What You Need to Know

Panic attacks aren't just in your head – they hijack your whole body. But they don't mean you're broken. They mean your brain has been running too many emergency drills.

Lesson 1: Your Fire Alarm is Faulty
Your brain isn't ruining your life – it's just *overactive* at threat detection.

TRY THIS: Next time panic strikes, instead of running, pause. Say (out loud or in your head): *'This is a false alarm. I am safe.'* The more you do this, the more your brain learns the difference between real danger and that burnt toast.

Lesson 2: People Won't Always Get It (and That Sucks, But It's Not Your Fault)
Being called 'dramatic', 'attention-seeking', or 'too sensitive' doesn't mean your experience isn't real. It just means they don't understand it.

TRY THIS: When someone minimises your panic, mentally hand them an invisible 'I don't get it' badge. Not everyone will understand and that's okay. You don't need their validation to know your experience is real.

REMINDER: You're not broken, you're learning and growing.

CHAPTER FOUR

The Fortress of Safety

"Avoidance builds walls around your life-strong enough to keep discomfort out, but also joy, freedom, and growth." (Sammy Barnett)

Ever felt like the outside world is just *too* much? Like, *'Nope, I'm out – I'll be in my blanket burrito if you need me.'*

Yeah? Same.

At first, it was a cosy retreat. A safe space. But soon, it became a no-surprises allowed fortress. Remote in one hand, dog by my side – only my most trusted allies allowed in.

It felt like control – until it wasn't.

The safety net I had built slowly tightened into a suffocating trap. Every escape route was mapped out ahead of time. No surprises. No curveballs. No situations that could trigger a panic attack.

That was the rule. That was survival.

But the real problem? I still had no answers.

I had no clue what was happening in my body, so avoiding everything felt like my only option. But anxiety wasn't a glitch – it had survival mode stuck on. And I had no idea how to switch it off.

It wasn't just screaming, *'RUN!'* for the fun of it.

It was a warning. A desperate signal that something inside me needed attention. That something deeper was going on.

But I didn't have the tools to decode it yet.

So instead of listening, I ran.

If a place, person, or activity had even the slightest chance of causing panic, it was a firm nope.

And the biggest *nope* of them all? School.

School? No Thanks

I was desperate. Not in a *'Please, Mum, I don't feel well'* kind of way. More like an *'I will absolutely swan-dive out of this moving car if you even think about stopping at the school gate'* kind of way.

The Fortress of Safety

And yes, I tried. More than once.

My mum was already juggling a divorce, financial stress and the chaos of single-parent life. And then she had me – her highly 'dramatic', would-rather-risk-traffic-than-face-social-anxiety child – throwing fuel onto the fire.

The school called my parents so often, I could have earned a VIP sick bay membership – and they might has well have had a permanent parking spot.

'Come collect Samantha.'
'She's in sick bay again.'
'She's refusing to go to class.'

The tone in their voice made me feel worse – like they thought I was faking it. But I wasn't sick. Not in the traditional sense. I spent more time in sick bay than I did in the classroom, curled up in the corner, pretending to have a stomach bug.

I was drowning in anxiety, just waiting for the moment I could retreat to my fortress of safety. But even inside my fortress, the weight of guilt followed me.

Avoidance with a Side of Guilt

My parents' relationship was already crumbling and I felt like I was making things worse.

'This is my fault', I told myself over and over again.

Anxiety has a way of making you believe you are the problem. But looking back, I see now – it wasn't *me* that was the burden. It was fear. My inability to process what was happening to me.

At the time, I couldn't separate the two. I *was* the fear. And I carried it like a personal failing.

At some point, the school must have realised I wasn't going at all anymore. So they got creative. They set up a space for me inside the office. A designated 'Sammy Space'.

Away from the crowds. Away from the judgment.

Clever.

It worked – for a while.

The Master of Avoidance

Avoidance didn't just stop at school. I took it to Olympic levels.

I wasn't just dodging uncomfortable situations – I was a full-blown escape artist.

I became *really* good at lying.

Not in an evil-genius, con-artist way. Just enough to escape any situation that felt remotely panic-inducing.

My escape plans became more elaborate by the day. And honestly? I should've been nominated for an award. Actually, scratch that

The Fortress of Safety

– I deserved my own *Netflix* documentary: *'Master of Avoidance: The Art of Making Up Plans That Don't Exist'*.

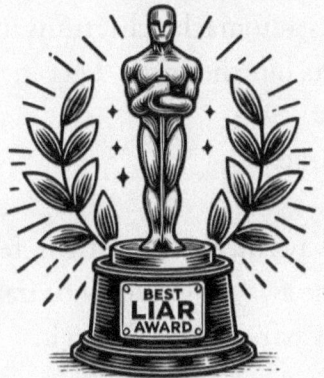

AND THE OSCAR FOR BEST LIAR GOES TO... SAMMY!

(For Outstanding Achievement in Avoiding Life)

Sammy would like to thank anxiety,
her overactive imagination and, of course,
her unwavering commitment to avoiding life at all costs.

Some of her most award-winning performances include:

I HAVE ASTHMA I CAN'T SWIM IN THE CARNIVAL!

THAT'S THE EXCURSION BUS, WE MISSED IT! OH WELL, NO SCHOOL

I SHOULD BE AT SCHOOL NOW, BUT I'M UNDER THE BED

I HAVE A HEADACHE AND NEED TO LAY IN THE QUIET ROOM ALL DAY

At first, they were harmless white lies. But in time, avoidance snowballs. Every excuse added another brick to my fortress.

Lying didn't help. It just proved to my brain that I couldn't handle life. And the more I avoided, the stronger that belief came.

The guilt gnawed at me like a slow-burning fire. My husband jokes that I could never get away with murder – my guilty conscience would betray me in minutes. We used to host poker tournaments before we had children, if I was dealt a pair of Aces, everyone knew. I couldn't fake it. My son is the same. Lying makes him physically ill. He gets a stomach-ache, turns into a nervous wreck and eventually blurts out the truth. I get it.

Because I am the same.

Lying made me feel awful. But back then, fear was bigger than guilt. If lying kept me away from the unbearable, all-consuming, I'm-dying-right-now panic, then I'd do it.

At that point, my number one value in life wasn't love, or joy, or adventure.

It was DEATH and avoiding it at all costs.

The irony? The harder I tried to stay safe, the smaller my world became.

The Fortress Becomes a Prison

Much of my life wasn't built around living – it was built around not dying. I wasn't obsessed with being healthy – I was obsessed with *not dying*.

The Fortress of Safety

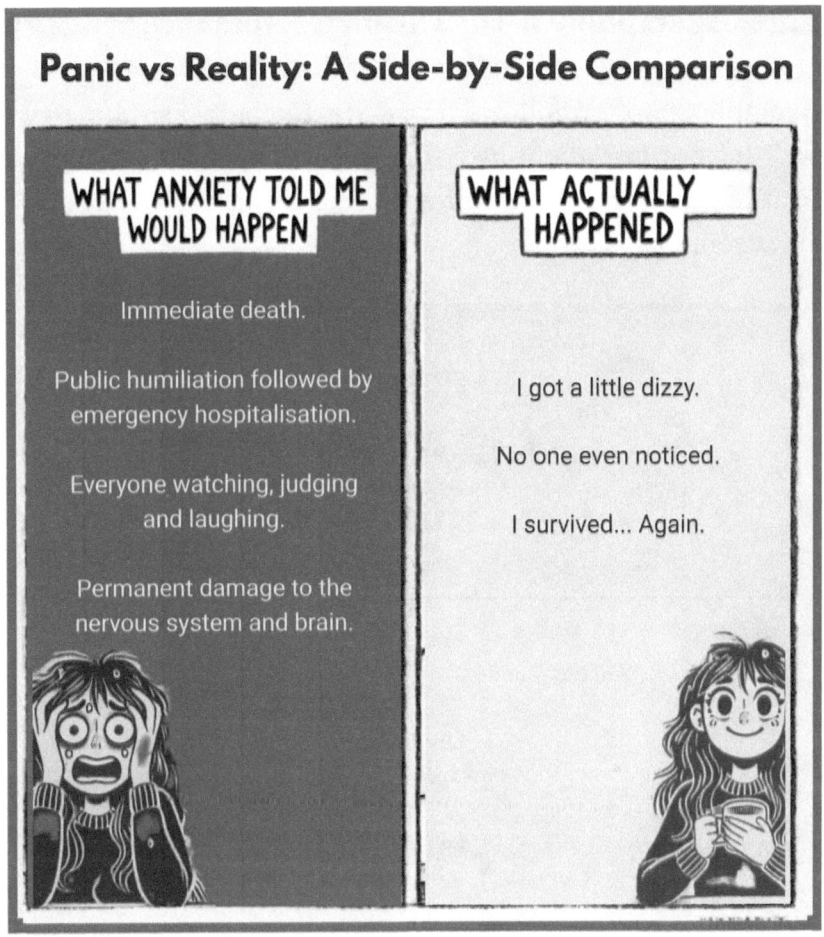

Anxiety was trying to keep me alive, but in the process, it was keeping me from truly living. That was the paradox: The very thing that was supposed to protect me was actually suffocating me.

At first, avoidance felt like control. It gave me the illusion of safety. But avoidance doesn't just stay in one place – it spreads. What started as skipping school and dodging social situations soon turned into something bigger.

Enter Agoraphobia: The Ultimate Avoidance Strategy

Agoraphobia often follows repeated panic attacks. (*Hi, that's me!*) It's not just about avoiding the outside – it's your brain treating the world like a war zone. For me, avoidance became an extreme sport.

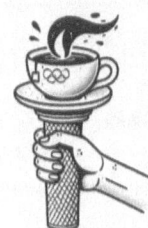

THE AGORAPHOBIA OLYMPICS

LEVEL 1:
You order takeout instead of picking it up.

LEVEL 2:
You time your food shop run to avoid human interaction.

LEVEL 3:
The delivery driver knocks. You hide behind the couch like a fugitive.

LEVEL 4:
You consider growing your own food to avoid supermarkets entirely.

LEVEL 5:
You've got a full doomsday bunker and now even the dog is concerned.

At first, it was great – no awkward small talk, no unexpected hugs. But eventually, even walking out to the letterbox felt impossible. My world kept shrinking.

Then came the side effects – weight loss, poor skin, exhaustion. I was constantly drained, living in a state of hypervigilance. My nervous system was fried just trying to keep me alive.

Looking back, I didn't realise anxiety wasn't just in my head – it was in my gut, too.

Anxiety was teaching me something else: that the body and mind are never separate. My body wasn't betraying me – it was responding exactly how it had been wired to respond. It wasn't failing me; it was trying to save me – just in all the wrong ways.

I wasn't eating properly. Chronic stress impacts digestion. When your nervous system is stuck in fight-or-flight mode, digestion takes a backseat. It's not just in your head – it's a real physiological response. Your body won't break down a sandwich properly if it thinks you're about to be eaten by a tiger.

I'll dive deeper into this later, but let's just say: Anxiety wasn't just messing with my mind – it was hijacking my gut, too.

Avoidance Makes Fear Bigger

Avoidance doesn't protect you. It isolates you.

I clung to the illusion that safety meant smallness, that comfort meant control. But every time I avoided something, I wasn't securing my freedom – I was reinforcing my captivity. My world kept getting smaller, but fear? It only grew.

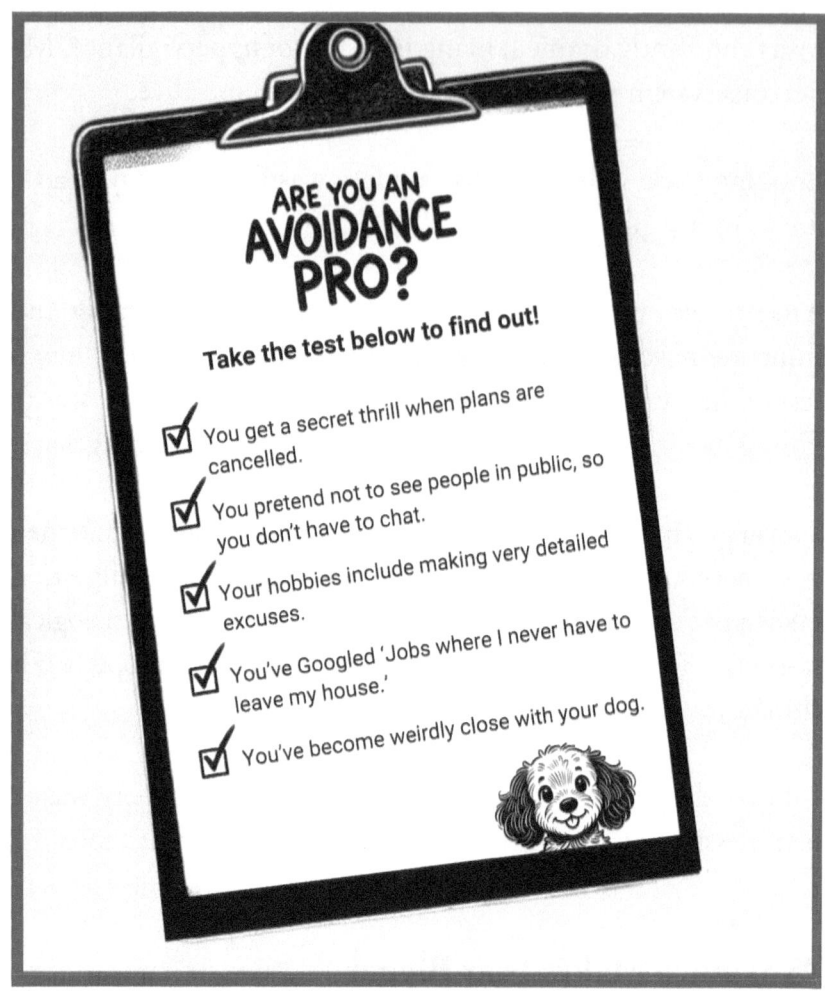

What I didn't know then was that fear fades when you face it – slowly, in small, manageable steps. That's the whole idea of exposure therapy – a method designed to retrain the brain and rebuild confidence.

But back then? The idea of leaning into fear instead of running from it sounded like absolute madness. I wasn't ready. Not yet.

The Fortress of Safety

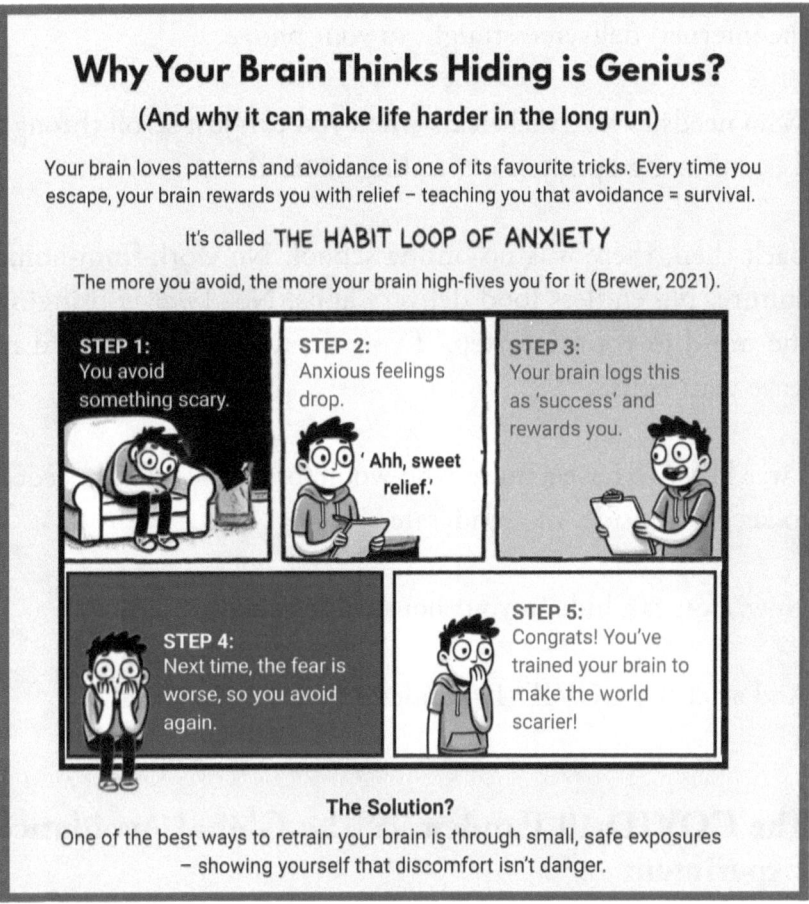

And let's be real – modern life now makes escaping ridiculously easy.

Avoidance in the 21st Century

Looking back, I see how technology has turned avoidance into an art form. In the 90s, if you wanted food, you had to actually go outside. Now? With the click of a button, you can get groceries, therapy and a whole new personality (courtesy of self-help podcasts and an overwhelming number of 'experts' on the internet) delivered straight to your phone.

Who needs to face their fears when you can just scroll through 47 conflicting opinions on healing instead?

Back then, there was no online school. No work-from-home culture. No endless food delivery apps. No *Amazon* bringing the world to your doorstep. If you wanted to live, you had to leave your house.

I was lucky to have a mum who would bring me what I needed to keep me inside, nice and 'safe.'

Now? You can hide in your house indefinitely.

And after the COVID-19 pandemic, a lot of people are.

The COVID-19 Pandemic: The Global Avoidance Experiment

When COVID-19 forced us inside, we weren't just avoiding the world – we were losing the skills to re-enter it.

I saw it in clinic – clients who once thrived in social settings now panicked over small talk, eye contact or even just sitting in a café alone.

Research shows that post-pandemic, social withdrawal is rising – especially in teens. A study found that excessive screen time is directly linked to increased anxiety and decreased face-to-face social skills (Twenge et al., 2020). The more we live online, the harder real-life interactions feel.

When I shut down my clinic and spent months working from home – no workshops, no speaking, no people – I told myself I was fine.

Then, when things started opening up, I had to relearn how to do things I used to do. Speaking on stages. Networking. Meeting new people.

It *should* have felt normal.

Instead, it felt like I was walking into a crowded room naked.

And I knew – that if I let avoidance win, I'd slip right back into my old fortress days.

And that's what happened to so many of us.

The pandemic didn't just lock us down – it rewired how we process safety and connection. Re-entering the world wasn't just about stepping outside. It was about relearning safety.

Melbourne took this to the extreme, where many people spent over 260 days inside – nearly a year of their lives. That wasn't just a lockdown. That was full-scale nervous system reprogramming. And we're seeing the fallout now. Children seem more reserved, struggling to engage. Parents? They can't shake the feeling that something still isn't right.

Because when your nervous system spends too long in survival mode, it forgets how to relax.

After years of having *'Stay inside, stay safe, stay away,'* drummed into you day after day, stepping back into the world doesn't just *feel* hard – it *is* hard.

But it's not just the isolation that contributed to this. It's what we consumed while we were isolated.

When we weren't out in the real world, experiencing life for ourselves, we were sitting in our fortresses, fed a 24/7 diet of fear:

- *The economy is collapsing!*
- *Violence is rising!*
- *Diseases are everywhere!*
- *Schools aren't safe!*
- *Climate catastrophe!*
- *The world is ending!*

We weren't just staying inside – we were consuming a constant stream of worst-case scenarios. And when your nervous system is already on high alert, that kind of input reinforces the idea that the world isn't safe. We were learning to fear it.

And now? Even though the doors are open, so many of us are still peeking out, wondering:

'Is it really safe out there?'

The Real Meaning of Safety

But here's what I've learnt: safety isn't staying home. Safety is learning that you can handle discomfort.

The Fortress of Safety

True safety isn't in avoidance – it's in trusting your own body again. The 'tiger' outside? He's not there to attack you – he's a messenger.

What if you listened? What if you learned his language?

What if – just maybe – you realised anxiety wasn't the villain you thought it was?

I wish I had known that then.

Instead, I spent years digging myself deeper into the avoidance hole, convinced it was the only way to survive.

But eventually, I climbed out.

And in the next chapters, I'll show you exactly how I did it.

Anxiety was never out to destroy me. It wasn't the enemy – it was the signal. The alarm bell I kept ignoring.

And the moment I finally listened?

That's when everything changed.

ANXIETY CHEAT SHEET:
What You Need to Know

The fortress you build for safety can quickly become your prison.

Lesson 1: Avoidance Doesn't Keep You Safe – It Keeps you Stuck
Avoidance doesn't just protect you from fear – it teaches your brain to fear more.

TRY THIS: Instead of asking, *'How can I avoid this?'* try, *'How can I make this feel 1% safer?'* Tiny steps build real confidence – not the illusion of it.

Lesson 2: Your Brain Thinks Hiding is a Genius Move (It's Not)
Avoidance rewards you with relief, so your brain keeps handing you more reasons to avoid. But the more you run, the scarier the world seems.

TRY THIS: When you catch yourself avoiding, pause. Say, *'Avoiding this makes fear bigger. Facing this makes fear smaller.'* Even if you do the thing for one minute, you've already disrupted the cycle.

REMINDER: The moment you stop avoiding? That's when fear finally starts to fade.

CHAPTER FIVE

Diagnosis: a Map or a Trap?

"Knowledge is power, but knowledge about yourself is self-empowerment."
(Dr Joe Dispenza)

I stumbled across a lifeline. It didn't make the panic disappear, but it gave me something I hadn't had in months: HOPE.

For so long, I had been drowning in confusion, convinced something was seriously wrong with me. This constant feeling of impending doom, of being different, of being broken – it followed me everywhere. But then, something changed.

I had an answer.

And great news...

I wasn't dying or going crazy!

After countless doctors' appointments, scans and specialists, most dismissed me as a hypochondriac or an overly worried child. Anxiety in children wasn't as widely recognised back then. Many didn't have the training or understanding as they do now. Doctors gave me two responses:

1. *It's just stress. Try relaxing!*
2. *Have you tried not being anxious?*

Ground-breaking. Truly life changing.

What I didn't know at the time was my mum was also experiencing panic attacks. She hid it well, not wanting to add to my worries. But looking back, I wonder – was I picking up on it anyway? Anxiety has a way of speaking in the silence, in the tension. Maybe I didn't have the words for it then, but I felt it.

Her own search for answers led her to a doctor who recommended a book: *Living With It: A Survivor's Guide to Overcoming Panic and Anxiety* by Bev Aisbett (1993).

She found it tucked away in a little bookstore, waiting for her – waiting for me.

It was one of the most life-changing books I had ever read.

The Power of a Name

For the first time, this thing had a name: anxiety and panic attacks.

I was then diagnosed with Generalised Anxiety and Panic Disorder – which basically meant my brain had decided to panic about the idea of a panic. A fun cycle of doom.

Getting this answer took time. Research shows girls are more likely to be dismissed as 'dramatic' or 'overreacting'. I wasn't imagining it.

How many other children are out there being told to 'calm down' when their nervous system is in a full-blown riot?

A diagnosis was a double-edged sword. It gave me a map – but it also felt like a label.

At first, my brain said, matter-of-factly, *'Well, you have anxiety and panic disorder, so this is just how you are now.'*

Fantastic.

Now I wasn't just anxious – I was *officially* anxious. Certified. Stamped and sealed.

But what if that wasn't true? What if anxiety wasn't trapping me?

What if, this whole time, it had been handing me the keys to understanding myself – and I just hadn't taken them yet?

I started asking different questions. *'If my brain had learnt to react this way... Could it unlearn it?'*

If anxiety had trained my brain for survival mode, could I train it for something else?

It's Just *Play-Doh*

Turns out, anxiety wasn't just about mindset – it was about mechanics.

What I *didn't* know then was that my brain wasn't set in stone – it was more like *Play-Doh*, thanks to neuroplasticity.

Diagnosis: a Map or a Trap?

✦ THE GREAT ✦
BRAIN
REWIRING PROJECT

Plot twist: My brain wasn't broken – it was just ridiculously over-trained in freak-out mode. Neuroplasticity is real. No magic switch, but with the right tools and repetition, we can retrain our brains.

Here's how the panic cycle works:

Feel anxious → FREAK OUT!! → Brain says 'Yep, this is dangerous!'

Repeat until fully convinced you're doomed.

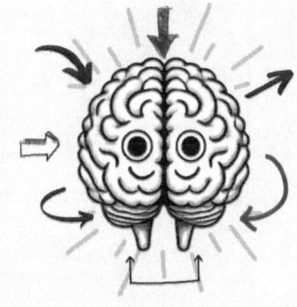

GOOD NEWS:
The same process that wired me for anxiety could be used to wire me out of it.

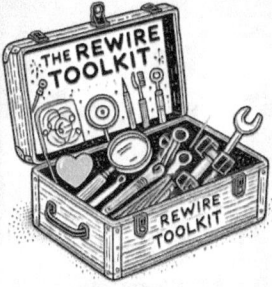

- Interrupt the cycle. (Stop. Breathe. Distract. There is no tiger.)

- Train the brain for chill mode. (Meditate, move and don't live off caffeine and sugar.)

- Make anxiety the test subject. (Stop fearing it, observe it. Hello, curiosity mode.)

Neuroscientist Norman Doidge dives deep into this in *The Brain That Changes Itself (2007)*, showing how we can reshape the brain with repetition, the right tools, and a little stubbornness.

For the first time, I realised my brain wasn't the enemy.

It had trained itself for survival mode.

Now, I had to train it in something new.

The First Book That Understood Me

Months had passed and the panic attacks hadn't stopped. But something was different.

I wasn't just experiencing them – I was starting to understand them.

Reading *Living with It* felt like looking into a mirror. The little girl drawn on the cover?

That was me!

The spiralling thoughts, the physical sensations, the fear that no one else could see? All there, laid out in simple language.

This book didn't talk AT me – it talked TO me. It didn't lecture or drown me in jargon or dismiss me as 'too young to understand'.

It was the first book I truly *understood* – and the first book that truly *understood me*.

Living With It didn't just help me – it helped the people around me too, with a guide for my family, friends and teachers.

Reading this made me feel less alone. Finally, there was something concrete to hand to the people in my life – a way to say, *'Here, this is what's happening inside me.'*

It showed me that the right support, from the right people, could make all the difference.

If you're a parent, teacher, or friend reading this – you don't have to fix it. Just being there, listening and giving space when needed can change everything for someone with anxiety and panic.

To this day, I've shared this exact book with family, friends and their children who are experiencing anxiety. And now? Full circle moment – I get to hand them *my* book, too.

Having something to *show* people meant I wasn't just being dramatic or overreacting, it gave my experience credibility.

And for a chronically anxious 11-year-old, that meant everything.

But knowing it was real wasn't enough – I wanted to know what to do with it.

Shifting from Fear to Curiosity

For the first time, I wasn't alone. I wasn't imagining it. And most importantly, what I was experiencing was real – and something I could work with.

But here's the thing: I didn't want to just *get through* it. Every book, doctor and conversation treated anxiety like something to *endure*. But what if that wasn't the point at all?

What if anxiety wasn't something to battle, supress or merely survive?

What if, all along, it was trying to teach me something?

Instead of fighting for control, what if we learnt to work with it? What if, rather than just managing anxiety, I could leverage it – turn it into a tool for growth.

That force building up inside me wasn't the enemy – it was energy. And once I learnt it's language, it stopped being something to fear.

That was my first big shift: turning fear into curiosity. If anxiety was speaking, I wanted to translate it.

This was the beginning of my deep dive into the human body – though I had no idea at the time how much it would shape my life. I don't do things halfway. If I was experiencing it, I needed to know it – inside and out.

My curiosity didn't stop at anxiety. It stretched to human behaviour, psychology – even true crime documentaries (which, yes, my husband finds a little concerning). But at the core of it all was the same question:

What makes people tick? What shapes our behaviours, fears and reactions?

I had spent years watching and learning from a distance. Now, for the first time, I was connecting the dots. My brain wasn't just reacting randomly – there was a pattern to it.

The First Taste of Power

My diagnosis didn't magically erase panic attacks, but something inside me had shifted. For the first time, I wasn't just experiencing anxiety – I was starting to understand it. And that tiny bit of knowledge?

It felt like power.

Anxiety wasn't random – it had rules.

It showed up when I wasn't prepared; when I felt watched, when I was caught off guard.

If it was going to keep me in full disaster-preparedness mode, I might as well become the CEO of Emergency Response.

Forget fire drills – I was running full-scale, military-level panic preparedness training.

Living with It listed places and situations that could set off panic attacks. So, in true 11-year-old obsessive fashion, I clung to that list like my life depended on it.

Behold: My personal guide to surviving the war zone that was school.

Anxiety: The Best TEACHER You Never Asked For

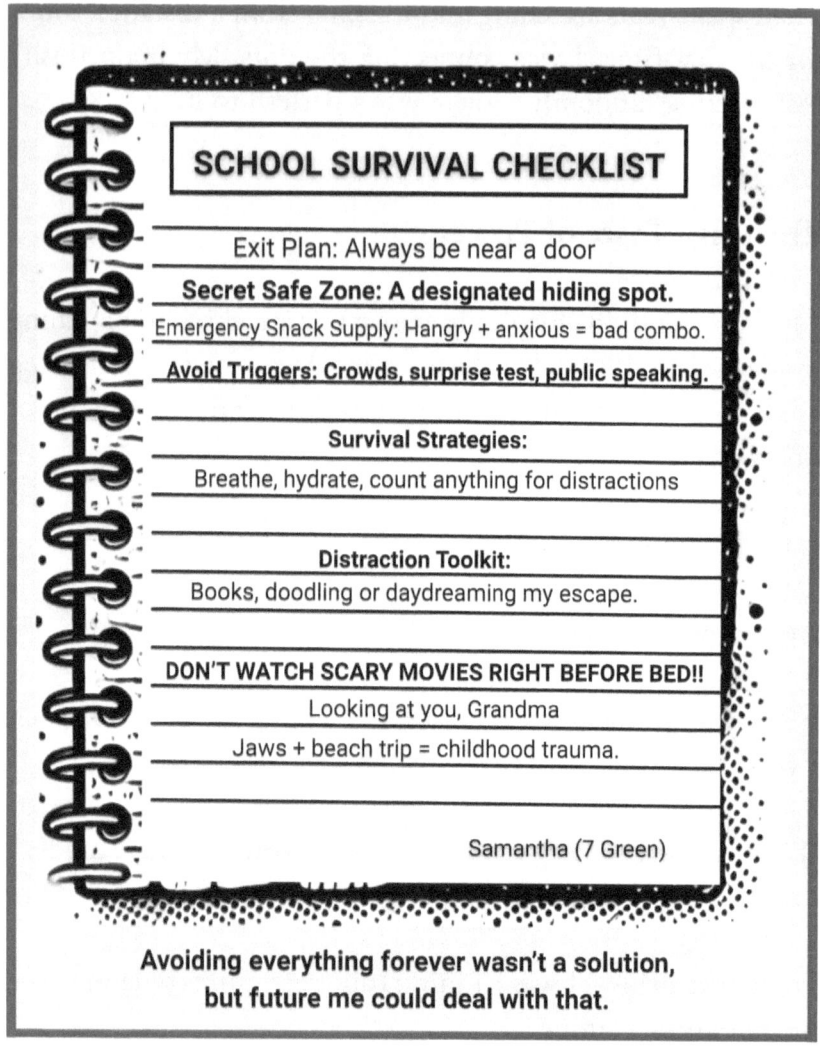

I had covered the external threats including strategically avoiding the worst possible seat in the classroom. But there was one thing I hadn't accounted for: the internal triggers.

Anxiety-Food Connection

What I didn't realise at the time? Anxiety wasn't just physical – it was chemical, too.

So, I started another list – because clearly, listing my fears wasn't enough. Now, I needed to know what food was fuelling them. *Living with It* had a list of some things already.

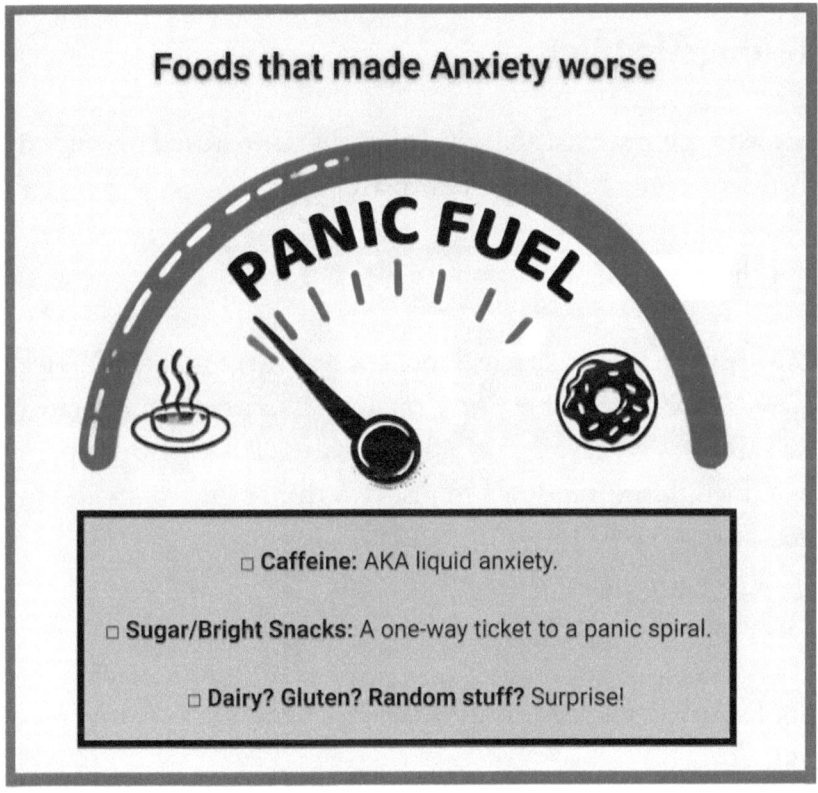

Research today digs deeper into the gut-brain connection, turns out I was onto something.

What I didn't know yet was that food wasn't just contributing to anxiety negatively – it could also make it better.

That connection? Yeah, I hadn't made it yet. Not even close.

Still, this list was all I had. My real deep dive into nutrition and anxiety would come later, but for now, I was clinging to what I could control.

Testing My Limits

Armed with my trusty survival checklist, I ventured beyond my fortress – ready to test my new plan.

But there was one tiny problem...

My list wasn't just a survival tool – it was turning into a *'How to Never Leave Your House Again'* manual. Every new 'safe' strategy was also a new reason to avoid something. If I kept this up, my world would shrink down to just two things: my room and my dog.

I needed a different approach.

So, I started experimenting with what I had learnt from *Living with It*.

What if I let the panic attacks come and go?

What if I just noticed them, instead of fighting them?

Diagnosis: a Map or a Trap?

I'd feel the panic creeping in, take a slow breath and remind myself:

'The world isn't disappearing. I'm just having a moment.'

This was the first time I really listened to my body.

We weren't exactly best friends yet, but I was trying. And I realised – reconnecting with myself was going to take time.

Had I ever been connected to myself? Or had I always been absent from my own body?

Tiny steps:

> ➢ Going to parties – but only with 'safe' people.
> ➢ Going to school – but giving myself permission to just breathe, stay quiet and not raise my hand.

I wasn't suddenly confident. I wasn't suddenly okay.

But I was learning.

I was testing the edge of my comfort zone – seeing how far I could push myself before the panic took over.

And then, I found something that pushed back – something that didn't trigger anxiety but made it subside.

My Happy Pace

I discovered something surprising. Sport made me feel amazing!

Even before the panic attacks started, movement had been calming – and I was *good* at it. Running, long jump – I could lose myself in the rhythm.

Before races, I was *wired* with nerves, but instead of shutting me down, it powered me up.

That ball of built-up energy? I used it to explode off the line.

I became age champion and was on my way to Districts and State. *Go me!*

Maybe anxiety wasn't something to escape – it was energy waiting to be used. Movement was medicine for me. My brain would stop spiralling mid-air, mid-jump.

My body was out here saying, *'Hey, I know how to fix this!'* all along.

Turns out, exercise is a secret nervous system hack. Who knew? Not me. If someone had told me movement was a cheat code for calming my brain, I might have skipped the whole *jumping-out-of-moving-cars* phase and just run alongside the car instead.

Exercise wasn't just clearing my head for fun – it was mixing up its own cocktail of feel-good chemicals.

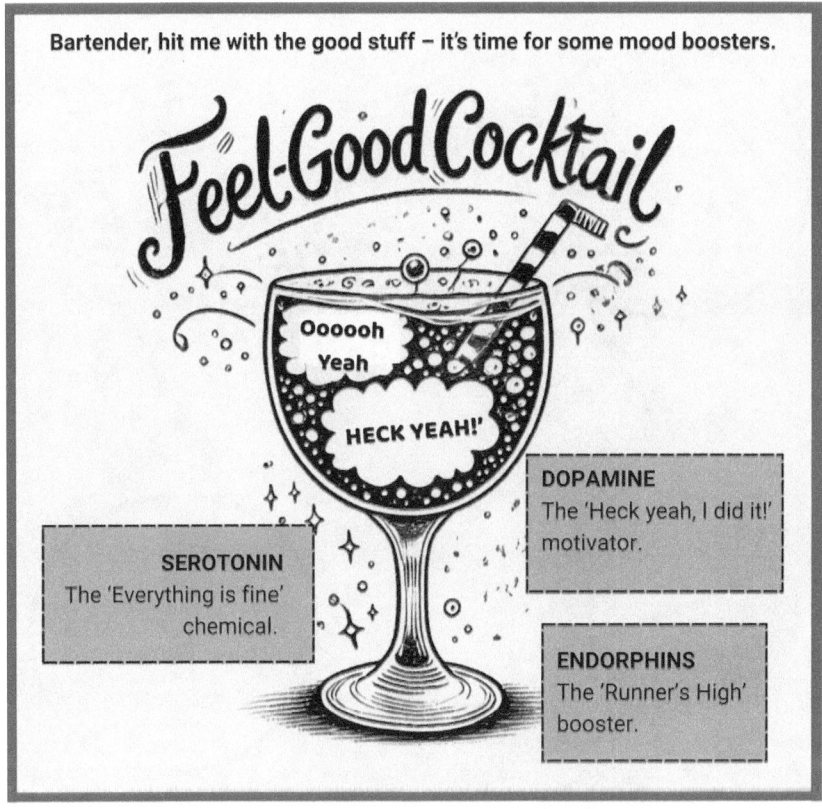

Exercise was hacking my brain for happiness.

What I didn't know at the time? These chemicals weren't just coming from my brain – they were being brewed mainly in my gut. And guess what? The bacteria living down there were running the whole operation.

(But I wouldn't figure that out until much later...and trust me, it changed everything.)

Anxiety: The Best TEACHER You Never Asked For

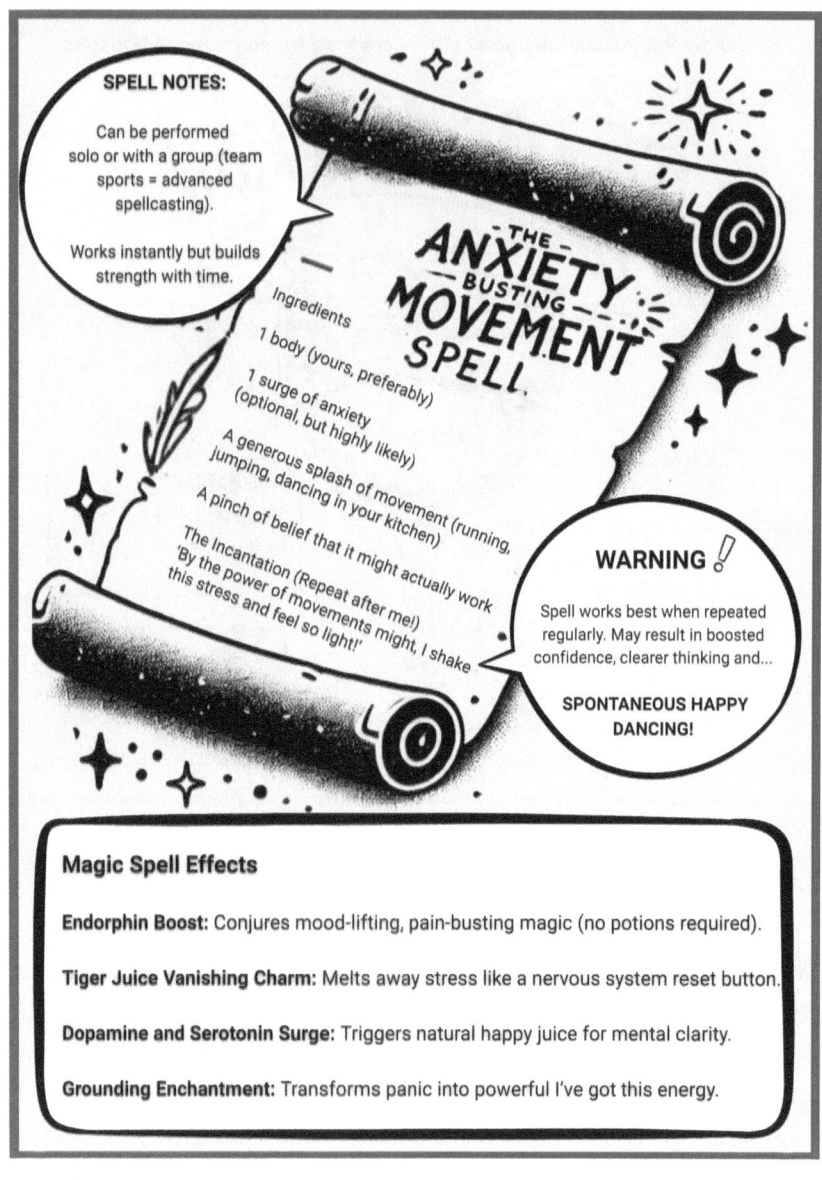

Exercise became a powerful tool for me, but I also know it's not a one-size-fits-all solution. For some, it's one piece of the puzzle – alongside therapy, medication, or other strategies. But for me? It was a game-changer.

Of course, like any good spell, you can overdo it. It would be years before I learnt too much of the wrong kind of exercise could actually spike that Tiger Juice even higher. Backfire alert!

But for now? I had found my happy pace. (See what I did there and you thought it was an error).

And then, something I never saw coming happened.

I became sports captain.

The shy anxious child. The one who faked sick days. The same girl who once had a full-blown existential crisis in the school bathroom.

That kid? Now leading war cries, making up chants, standing in front of the entire school – with teammates, of course.

What a plot twist.

How? Because the moment I learnt I *wasn't dying*, I knew I had to start *living*.

But I wasn't reckless about it. I tested my limits in places where I already felt strong. Sport had structure. Sport had rules. Sport had cheerleaders – people literally shouting encouragement at me. It was the perfect space to start pushing myself.

And something shifted.

I wasn't just moving my body – I was learning how to trust it. To work with it. To listen to it.

The Beginning of Everything

I had no idea that my obsession with understanding my own mind and body would shape my future.

Beneath all the experimenting, a new version of me was forming – not just surviving but learning. Anxiety was no longer just an enemy – it was becoming a teacher.

But growth came with grief. I mourned the version of me that once moved through the world without scanning for escape routes, without second-guessing every sensation.

Still, with every bit of knowledge I gained, something stronger than fear emerged: HOPE.

And one day, I could teach others to find it, too.

ANXIETY CHEAT SHEET: What You Need to Know

Getting diagnosed with anxiety and panic disorder felt like a double-edged sword – it gave me answers, but it also made me feel like this was now my whole identity.

Lesson 1: A Diagnosis is a Map, Not a Trap
Diagnosis can feel like a trap if we let it define us. But really, it's just the first step.

TRY THIS: Instead of thinking, *'I have anxiety, so this is just how I am,'* reframe it: *'Now that I know what this is, I can learn how to work with some of the information around it.'* Labels don't limit you – how you respond to them does.

Lesson 2: Movement is Medicine (and I Accidentally Discovered It)
Turns out, exercise wasn't just making me good at sport – it was rewiring my nervous system.

TRY THIS: Feeling anxious? Move. It doesn't have to be a marathon – shake it out, dance like a maniac in your kitchen, or go for a quick walk. Your brain thrives on movement and so does your nervous system.

REMINDER: A diagnosis isn't a cage – it's a key.

CHAPTER SIX

Chasing Validation

*"When you do not seek or need approval,
you are at your most powerful."*
(Caroline Myss)

Avoidance was my greatest coping mechanism, but it cost me my identity, confidence and connection. I could handle small steps – until discomfort knocked.

I would soon realise anxiety wasn't just discomfort – it was a teacher.

It wasn't pushing me.

It was pointing out where I needed to grow.

Sure, I could leave my house – under carefully controlled conditions. I had designed a life I could tolerate, not one I could thrive in.

I had a mental list of *no-go zones*.

- ➤ Concert? Too many eyes on me.
- ➤ Social events? Only if I had a security blanket.

My world was structured around what I *could* handle. I 'managed' anxiety with shallow breathing and sheer hope.

Worry lingered like a black cloud – not always there but never gone.

And when the discomfort became unbearable? I found another crutch: Validation.

The only time I wasn't worried was when people told me I was doing great. If I couldn't feel safe in myself, I could at least feel safe in their approval.

By high school, boys entered the mix. At first, the attention felt good – I felt seen.

But attention isn't respect and desire isn't value.

As Hank Ketcham says, *"Flattery is like chewing gum. Enjoy it briefly, but don't swallow it."*

Scrolling for Self-Worth

Validation seeking doesn't disappear – it evolves. Then, it was boys. Now? Likes, comments and follower counts.

Social media has put validation seeking on steroids. And it's not just teens.

I met so many women in my clinic – successful, accomplished – still caught in the loop, believing their worth depended on how others perceived them.

We think we grow out of it. Do we? Or do we just get better at masking it?

Every like, every *'You look amazing, hun!'* triggers a small dopamine hit – the brain's reward signal. And just like any addict, one hit is never enough.

Before you know it, you're refreshing your feed like a slot machine, waiting for another hit of *'You're enough.'*

I am grateful I didn't grow up in the social media era. But even without it, the pressure to be 'enough' never really left. It just changed shape.

But here's the thing – when I stopped chasing validation, I didn't find freedom. I found another kind of cage.

Fading into the Background

Society's unspoken rulebook told me to be smaller, softer, agreeable. I toned down my style, my voice, my presence – because blending in felt safer. I disappeared into beige and grey.

Recently, a friend took one look at my closet and said, *'Are you okay?'*

I felt exposed. I was dressing to fade into the background.

Sometimes the way we dress is a cry for help in fabric form. If I could hide in plain sight, maybe I wouldn't have to face the parts of myself I was too scared to confront.

The next day, I bought a bright, orange dress. It felt like a neon sign. But for the first time in years, I didn't want to disappear.

As I got older, I craved solitude. Not loneliness – just the comfort of being with someone who didn't expect anything from me. Enter: dogs.

Dogs don't judge. Cats do – aggressively. Except Freddy, the Sphinx cat. He is bald, so I think he has his own insecurities.

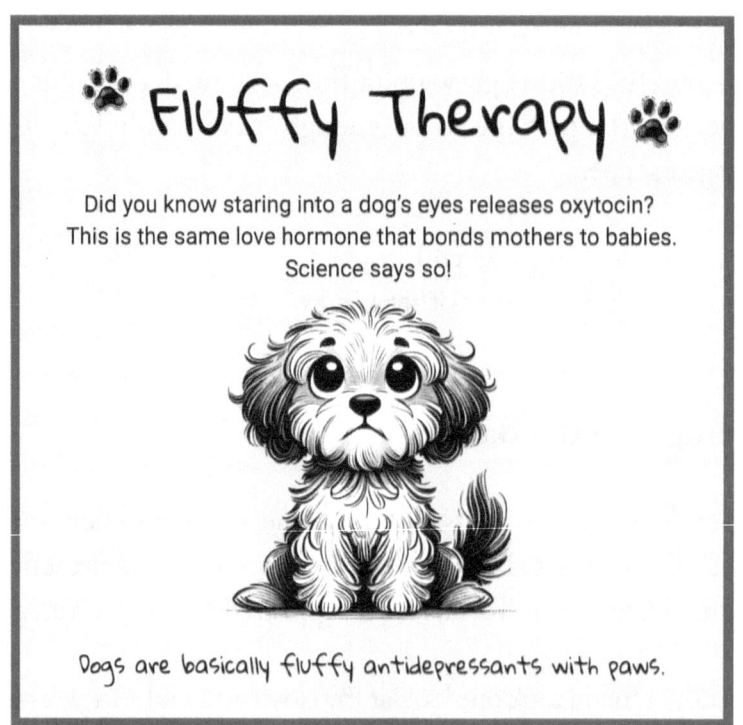

As much as I found comfort in animals, I knew real safety couldn't come from hiding in solitude – or in a dog's unconditional love. At some point, I had to feel safe in myself.

For years, I stayed in the shadows. I dimmed myself down so I wouldn't steal the light from others. But now? I take up space. I light up rooms instead of shrinking in them.

True acceptance doesn't come from others (or your pets). It comes from within. And once you realise this, the world stops feeling so heavy.

From Invisible to Seen

By my mid-teens, panic attacks had slowed to once a week. Progress, sure, but I was still waiting for the next one to strike.

Life wasn't slowing down for me. My mum was working full-time, my dad had moved away and money was tight. I had to step up. There were no hand-outs for me – just work. A lot of it.

Three jobs, to be exact:

> - A waitress – forcing social skills!
> - Receptionist – first nightmare boss, thankfully, I had earned my black belt in People Pleasing.

And then, my wildest job at that point?

A clown! Yes, a literal clown.

Oddly, kids felt safer than adults. The adults, however, had left positive feedback, saying how interactive and fun I was and their children looked forward to seeing me.

Me – the girl who avoided, who shrank herself, who lived in the shadows.

For years, I had convinced myself that blending in was best for survival. That the less I spoke, the safer I was. That invisibility was protection. But here I was, in a ridiculous clown costume, fully seen – and not just tolerated, but celebrated.

Had I been wrong?

It was in these little moments I was starting to push back against anxiety. Not in some grand, movie-worthy epiphany, but in the simplest way: By showing up, making kids laugh and letting myself take up space – even in a costume.

And maybe... I didn't have to live so small.

Hormones Gone Wild

Just as I was feeling a tiny bit in control, my body had other plans.

Enter: Hormones.

A full-blown production where my brain, body and emotions were now being directed by The Hormonal Drama Club.

While I got my period quite young, things didn't start getting really wild until high school. Nothing says *'Welcome to Womanhood'* like bike pants and a high jump bar.

Early puberty is linked to increased anxiety. And looking back, it makes so much sense. The sudden surges of oestrogen and cortisol (aka Tiger Juice) created a hormone-fuelled storm inside me. Rapid changes – physically, emotionally, mentally – while my nervous system was already on high alert? Recipe for disaster.

Throw in some progesterone (or the lack thereof) and suddenly I wasn't just dealing with anxiety – I was dealing with a full-scale hormonal rebellion.

Puberty didn't care I was already drowning in overthinking. It crashed in. Zero warning, no script and a cast of unpredictable hormones determined to take centre stage.

Anxiety: The Best TEACHER You Never Asked For

THE HORMONAL DRAMA CLUB

starring <u>Oestrogen</u> and <u>Progesterone</u>.

The high school drama you never signed up for – Prepare for mood swings, plot twists and a backstage crew of hormones working overtime!

Beware of Oestrogen Tantrums
These Divas take their job very seriously.

The Snack Table Scandal
Your liver's busy dealing with excess toxins to remove Oestrogen. So instead of exiting gracefully, they stay past cue. ENCORE!

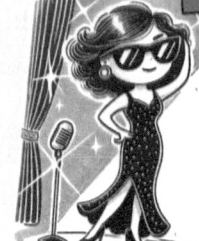

OESTROGEN – The Divas Who Don't Know When to Leave

Role? Set the stage for pregnancy. Roll out a plush, velvety red carpet (aka your uterine lining).

Xenoestrogens: The Stunt Doubles
Think plastics. They sneak in, causing chaos and confusion.

Gut Issues: The Stage Crew on Strike
Your gut should escort excess Oestrogen off set. But if digestion is sluggish, they refuse to leave the dressing room. Cue bloating, PMS and emotional meltdowns.

The problem?
They go overboard – building a five-star luxury hotel for a VIP guest who never shows. And when it's time to tear it down? Let's just say... it can get messy (aka the bleed).

Stress: Stage Fight
Cortisol crashes the scene, Oestrogen panic and suddenly they're running the whole show. The result? Mood swings, bloating and a period straight out of a horror movie.

Keep Oestrogen in Check!! A little makes the show amazing. Too much? Total disaster.

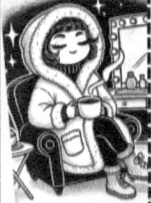

PROGESTERONE - The Chill Sidekicks

Supposed to keep things calm in the second half of your cycle. These laid-back besties make sure you sleep, feel balanced and don't murder anyone. But if you're too busy making cortisol, they won't show.

NOTE...if Oestrogen steal the spotlight (bloody bitches), progesterone struggle to get a word in. Think rage, anxiety, sleepless nights and sugar cravings (cue the sudden need for chocolate and an irrational hatred of everyone).
DON'T TOUCH ME!

Plot Twists

Puberty brings a surprise twist of emotions and hormones have no idea what they're doing.

Cortisol storms the set, making anxious feelings worse.

Oestrogen and blood sugar drops before your period, dragging serotonin (happy hormone) down with it. Hello sudden sadness, irritation and that urgent need for hot chips and chocolate.

Get ready for an emotional ride that explains why your hormones have a starring role in your mental health drama!

Hormones don't stop controlling the show after puberty. And for me? They were just warming up.

Puberty might be the opening act, but what happens when the curtain falls? Do the hormones take a graceful bow and exit stage left?

Yeah, no. They stick around – sometimes with an encore you didn't ask for.

Hormone Hangover

Once puberty settles (and your hormones stop acting like chaotic theatre kids in a never-ending improv show), your cycle should stabilise – but that doesn't always mean everything magically balances itself out.

For some, the drama quietens down. For others? Heavy periods, mood swings and a body still trying to figure itself out.

And if heavy periods stick around, it can lead to ongoing issues like low iron – which is where things start getting even trickier. In my clinic, low iron was one of the most common deficiencies I saw in menstruating women. And here's the thing: Low iron isn't just about feeling tired.

It's tied to anxiety, too.

Yep, it's a double whammy! When iron levels drop, your body struggles to transport oxygen properly. This can make you feel wired but exhausted, breathless, dizzy and of course…more anxious!

The fix? A quality iron supplement to boost levels quicker, while at the same time working on WHY the bleed was so heavy in the first place. And this brings us to 'The Pill'.

The quick fix to 'regulate' things.

But does it really solve the problem? Or just cover it up?

Ahhh, The Pill.

A tiny tablet that turned me into a raging hormonal monster. If there ever was something that showed me the power of hormones, it was this.

I was put on The Pill at 15. I was a total bitch on The Pill.

For some, it's life changing. For others (like me), it's a hormonal rollercoaster. I've met countless women struggling with mood swings, gut issues and depression – never considering their birth control might be the culprit. Instead of getting answers, they were handed more prescriptions.

Madness, right?

The Magical Pill:
A Quick Fix or Mood-Hacker

Once upon a time, there was a tiny, mystical tablet promising to vanish period problems, clear skin and make cycles 'regular'.

But here's the catch: Magic always comes with a price.

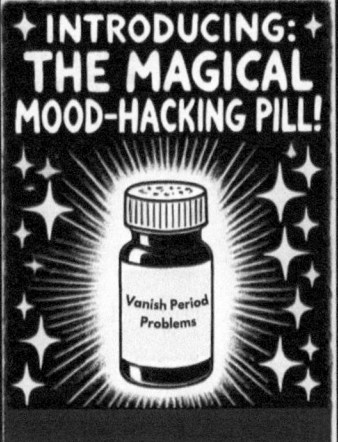

How Does the 'Magic' work?

The Pill doesn't fix your hormones – it shuts them down completely. No ovulation means:

- No natural progesterone (your chill hormone).
- Oestrogen stays low, so your uterine lining never gets a chance to build up.
- Your monthly 'bleed' isn't even a real period – it's just a withdrawal from synthetic hormones. (A hormonal illusion, if you will.)
- Less uterine lining = less to shed = lighter bleeds. **MAGIC!**

More like a smoke and mirrors trick.

But What's Hiding Under the Spell?

B Vitamin Heist → The Pill steals B6, B12 and folate – the VIPs of serotonin production (aka your happy hormones).

Inflammation Potion → Can leave you feeling bloated, fatigued, or just 'off.'

Gut Disruption → Since up to 95% of serotonin is made in the gut, messing with bacteria can trigger anxiety and low mood.

Mood Mysteries → Research shows women on The Pill have a higher risk of depression – some feel emotionally muted, others notice anxious feelings creeping in for no reason.

Is The Pill a Villain or Just a Trickster?

For some, it works like a quick-fix spell. But for others, it's like putting a glamour charm over the real problem – hiding symptoms instead of fixing them.

Because in the end, **real magic comes from knowing how your body actually works.**

Breaking the Spell

I was on The Pill until I was 22 – it was seven years of hell.

My body had no clue how to process synthetic hormones. I was already struggling to absorb B vitamins and The Pill just poured fuel on the fire.

When I finally listened and stopped taking The Pill? The anger that had been running through my veins, the sudden mood swings, irrational outbursts? They faded. It was like someone turned the volume down. Things that used to send me into a blind fury no longer registered.

My husband was never going to let me take The Pill again – not just for my sake but his!

The truth is, The Pill wasn't the only thing keeping me from feeling like myself. I had spent so many years trying to 'manage' anxiety, shrink myself, avoid discomfort and sidestep anything that felt like a risk. And in doing so?

I missed out on a lot.

Watching From the Sidelines

The more I avoided, the more I lost pieces of myself.

High school was a blur of fear. I watched others around me *achieve* while I sat in bitterness. Stuck in the constant cycle of fear and self-doubt. And I *hated* that everyone else was moving forward.

The more I indulged in negative emotions, the stronger those pathways were becoming. That bitterness made me a not-so-nice person for a time. I was negative. Jealous. Judgmental.

I see it in women now – 40s, 50s and 60s – who feel they missed their chance in life.

If you're reading this thinking, *'Yep, that's me,'* trust me, I see you. This isn't where your story ends. I have met and worked alongside many women who reclaimed who they are. The trajectory of their life has changed well into their 70s.

It's never too late.

Bitterness is often an unmet desire in disguise. Other times, it's rooted in old wounds we haven't fully processed. Either way, it has something to teach us – if we're willing to listen.

Instead of resenting people who have what you want – learn from them. And don't let those anxious feelings stop you in your tracks. Anxiety isn't just fear – it's a map. It can point toward the things you deeply care about, the places where growth is waiting. Tap into it. Ask it what it's trying to teach you.

Because at the end of the day, anxiety never actually took anything from me. I did that all by myself.

But now? I'm taking it all back.

Reclaiming Me

Validation stole years from me. I refuse to let it steal more.

So, I'm taking it all back.

I'm taking back my voice – because quiet didn't allow the self-expression I craved.

I'm taking back my body – because shrinking didn't keep me safe, it kept me disconnected.

I'm taking back my joy – because I don't need permission to feel light and free.

I'm taking back my choices – because fear-based decisions are just invitations to grow.

I left these behind.

Now? I'm picking them back up.

For years, I let fear and the need for approval dictate my choices. I shrank myself to fit into a world that never asked me to. But the truth is – no one was stopping me from living, except me.

The validation I chased, the avoidance I mastered, they weren't protecting me. They were trapping me.

Anxiety wasn't the enemy.

It wasn't a flashing neon sign warning me to hide – it was a quiet guide whispering, *'There's more for you.'*

And now? I'm finally starting to pay attention.

ANXIETY CHEAT SHEET:
What You Need to Know

True validation isn't given – it's reclaimed.

Lesson 1: External Validation is a Bottomless Pit
Validation is craving, not a cure.

TRY THIS: Instead of wondering, *'What will they think?'* ask *'What do I think?'* Approval means nothing if it costs your authenticity.

Lesson 2: Shrinking Yourself Doesn't Keep You Safe – It Keeps You Small
Shrinking didn't protect me – it just kept me disconnected. Blending in wasn't survival – it was self-abandonment.

TRY THIS: Notice where you're toning yourself down to be accepted. Are you dressing, speaking, or living for others' comfort at the expense of your own? Start with one small act of self-expression – even if it's just wearing the damn orange dress.

REMINDER: You don't have to prove your worth to take up space in this world.

CHAPTER SEVEN

Fighting the 'Monster'

"The only way to tame the monster is to stop running and finally face it." (Unknown)

There comes a time when hiding is no longer an option. My hands trembled as I gripped my tiny shield, stepping out into the darkness. Courage isn't about being fearless – it's about moving forward despite the fear.

Fear ruled my life. I thought I was protecting myself, but really, I was shrinking my world. I convinced myself I was growing – but only in the places that felt safe. The parts of me that were withering. Those were the ones I needed to step into.

But stepping into them? Terrifying. Like accidentally liking someone's photo from 2012 while deep in stalking their *Facebook* session. Yeah, done that. And no, there's no recovery from it.

Anxiety had been screaming at me for years and for the longest time, I thought it was just there to torment me. But eventually, I realised it wasn't just yelling – it was trying to tell me something. I wasn't the problem. It was pointing me toward the problem.

I knew what I needed to do. I had to face my fears. But knowing and doing?

Two very different things.

I wasn't ready. But here's the thing – no one ever feels ready. You just do it.

Most of the big changes I had to make weren't because I wanted to. They happened out of necessity – financial stability, survival, safety. Every time, I had to step off a metaphorical bridge, not knowing where I'd land. I had to fall first. And only then did I learn: *The net appears after the leap, not before.*

Growing up in an unstable financial situation, you realise quickly – you don't get the luxury of waiting. You just jump. Not just for yourself, but for the people you love.

Acting My Way Into Confidence

This necessity to act despite fear laid the foundation for building confidence. People see me now and say, '*Wow, you're so confident! You get on stage, you speak, you do all these things.*'

The truth is, I still feel all the feels. But I do it anyway.

Those feelings? They've just been rerouted.

Instead of fear, I feel excitement.

Instead of dread, I feel anticipation.

You build confidence by stepping into roles you never thought you could handle.

But first, I had to get past my brain's dramatic tendencies.

Anxiety: The Best TEACHER You Never Asked For

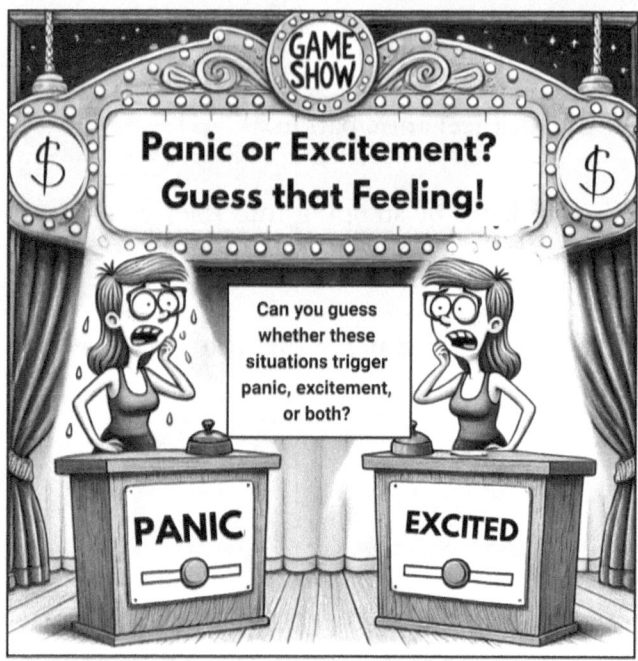

1. You're about to give a big speech. Your heart is pounding, palms sweaty. You feel like throwing up. **PANIC or EXCITEMENT?**

Answer: BOTH! Your brain processes them the same way. But if you reframe it as, 'I'm excited to share my ideas!' you actually perform better.

2. You're about to get on a rollercoaster. Your stomach drops, legs feel wobbly. Your breathing speeds up. **PANIC or EXCITEMENT?**

Answer: BOTH! That's just your body gearing up for action. Reframe it: 'This is a thrill, not a threat!'

3. You get a text at 2am from your son saying, 'Come quick.' Your heart pounds, throat tightens. You can't think straight. **PANIC or EXCITEMENT?**

Answer: PANIC! Unless you're about to become a Grandma! That's exciting! Or is it?

Your brain is like that one overdramatic friend who hears 'big life change' and immediately screams, 'WE'RE GONNA DIE!'

But panic and excitement feel the same in your body. Your heart races. Your palms sweat. Your stomach does that weird rollercoaster drop.

The Jedi Mind Trick

Turns out, your brain is kind of gullible. Studies suggest that if you tell yourself, *'I'm excited,'* instead of, *'I'm anxious,'* your brain just…rolls with it. A Harvard study found that reframing nerves as excitement actually helped people perform better (Brooks, 2014).

And me? I took that research years later and ran with it – straight into the most ridiculous confidence hack ever.

I Jedi-mind tricked myself into thinking that standing in front of hundreds of people with a microphone was a good thing. I used the force. It's the hack of the century.

    1: Yell *'I'M EXCITED!'* at yourself repeatedly.

    2: Your brain reluctantly agrees.

    3: The neighbour shows up with champagne, assuming you got engaged, won the lottery, or finally learnt how to fold that fitted sheet.

But hey – you're pumped instead of panicked. You just put a fun party hat on your fear. Woohoo!

Using the Jedi-mind trick was great in theory, but I needed a way to practice confidence in real life. Saying, *'I'm excited!'* in my mirror was one thing, but I needed something bigger – something that would actually force me to step into discomfort.

Enter: Acting classes.

My New Hobby

When I started dating my husband, I noticed he had all these hobbies and I had…none. My hobby was not dying. But after all this work on rewiring my anxious brain, I figured it was time to try something new – something just for me.

For some reason, I landed on acting.

It made *no* sense. I had spent my life disappearing, avoiding situations where I could be seen or judged. But deep down, I wanted to feel comfortable in my own skin.

I'd heard of '*fake it 'til you make it,*' but I didn't believe in faking anything. Then I came across something better: '*Be it until you see it!*'

That became my new motto!

The brain doesn't always know the difference between real and imagined experiences. If I could *act* confident, maybe – just maybe – I could *become* confident. Neuroplasticity, right?

So, I did something completely out of character. I signed up for an acting class. If I was going to trick my brain into believing I had confidence, I needed a stage to practice on.

And that's when Keanu Reeves appeared.

Not literally – unfortunately – but spiritually.

Keanu looked at me, all wise and smouldering and said, '*Fear is an illusion, Samantha.*'

Fighting the 'Monster'

Then he handed me a script with no words on it.

I stared at the blank page.

He nodded. I nodded back.

This was it. Keanu had spoken. I had no choice but to improvise my way to victory.

Cut to reality: My first class was full-scale disaster.

Sweaty palms. Heart racing. Brain screaming in *SpongeBob SquarePants*' voice, '*WE'RE GONNA DIE IN FRONT OF ALL THESE PEOPLE!*'

I opened my mouth to speak…and my brain immediately deleted all knowledge of the English language. Just poof. Gone. I was standing there, blinking in Morse code, waiting for someone to save me.

But I didn't die.

Funny that.

The fear was in my head the whole time.

And something weird happened – nobody cared. Not even Keanu. Nobody was laughing at me. In fact, they were supportive. The only person judging me? Me.

Turns out, fear is just a voice. Not reality. The only way to grow is to walk into it. That became another new motto: '*Feel the fear and do it anyway.*'

Anxiety: The Best TEACHER You Never Asked For

But here's the thing – why does fear feel so real when logically, I know I'm safe?

THE ANXIETY TIMES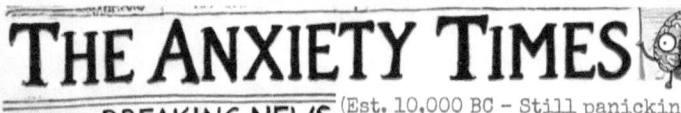

(Est. 10,000 BC – Still panicking today)

BREAKING NEWS
ANXIETY FOUND USING OUDATED MANUAL!

Experts confirm anxiety has been running on a perfectly designed but sometimes overprotective survival system. Despite modern advancements, the Caveman Brain Security System refuses to upgrade.

Outdated Operating System Discovered

A recent investigation into the Limbic System – home of the emotional brain – has revealed shocking inefficiencies.

Head of Security

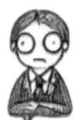

The Limbic System (aka prehistoric security guard)

Mission: Keep you alive.
Flaw: Can't tell the difference between actual danger and mildly inconvenient situations.

Staff Under Review

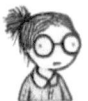 **Amygdala**

Job Title: Chief Alarm Sounder

Performance Review: Hits panic button way too often, mistaking work emails for tiger attacks.

Official Statement: 'Danger is danger! It's my job to FREAK OUT!'

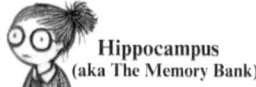 **Hippocampus**
(aka The Memory Bank)

Job Title: Head of Emotional Archives

Performance Review: Files all scary experiences as 'life threatening' with zero expiration.

Recent Incident: Declared public speaking as equally terrifying as being chased by a tiger.

LOGIC DEPARTMENT CALLS FOR <u>URGENT</u> UPGRADE

The Prefrontal Cortex (aka The Thinking Brain) – the newest department in the brain – is demanding an immediate manual rewrite.

Job Title: Head of logic, problem-solving and rational thinking.

Official Statement: 'We are NOT in the Stone Age anymore! My department is working overtime trying to teach the Limbic System that public speaking is NOT the same as being chased by a tiger. But hey, old habits die hard.'

From Caveman Brain to Hollywood (Sort Of)

This whole 'brain still thinks I'm a caveman' thing explained a lot.

It wasn't that I was actually bad at acting – it was that my prehistoric security system had me convinced I'd be alone and eaten alive if I embarrassed myself.

So, I played it safe.

I wasn't diving into lead roles. My acting was *decent*, but I was mainly an extra in films – just blending into the background. I already knew how to do that. It was fun. Easy money. Sitting in a resort, pretending to sip cocktails.

Then came a moment I *didn't* see coming – an actual hero role in a movie starring Ethan Hawke! I was going to be one of the 'Daywalkers' in his vampire film. Exciting right!?

A hero role meant I wasn't just in the background – I'd actually be *in* the scene. Maybe even say a line.

And what did I do?

I turned it down!

Why? Because I had already booked tickets to *The Simpsons Movie* in Gold Class and apparently, that was more important. My 22-year-old-self made that call.

Yep. That was my big Hollywood moment. My chance to be a hero. My moment in the spotlight. And what did I do? I sacrificed it for a cartoon man who eats donuts.

Doh!

Somewhere, alternate-universe-me is sipping matcha with Meryl. *This* me? Sitting in a recliner, covered in Gold Class popcorn crumbs.

Looking back, I can't help but wonder – was that just bad timing or was it self-sabotage? Was I avoiding something bigger?

At the time, I didn't think much of it. I was enjoying myself. I met incredible people in the acting world – people who seemed confident but were actually feeling all the same nerves I was. They weren't fearless. They were just showing up, over and over, until confidence became their reality.

Just like me, they were *acting* their way into bravery.

But I still didn't get it. I still thought I had to fight this thing inside me. I hadn't yet realised it wasn't my enemy. I wasn't learning from anxiety – I was still trying to eliminate it.

And, in my mind, I was winning.

But here's what I know now: Anxiety isn't something you defeat. It's something you can train.

Fighting the 'Monster'

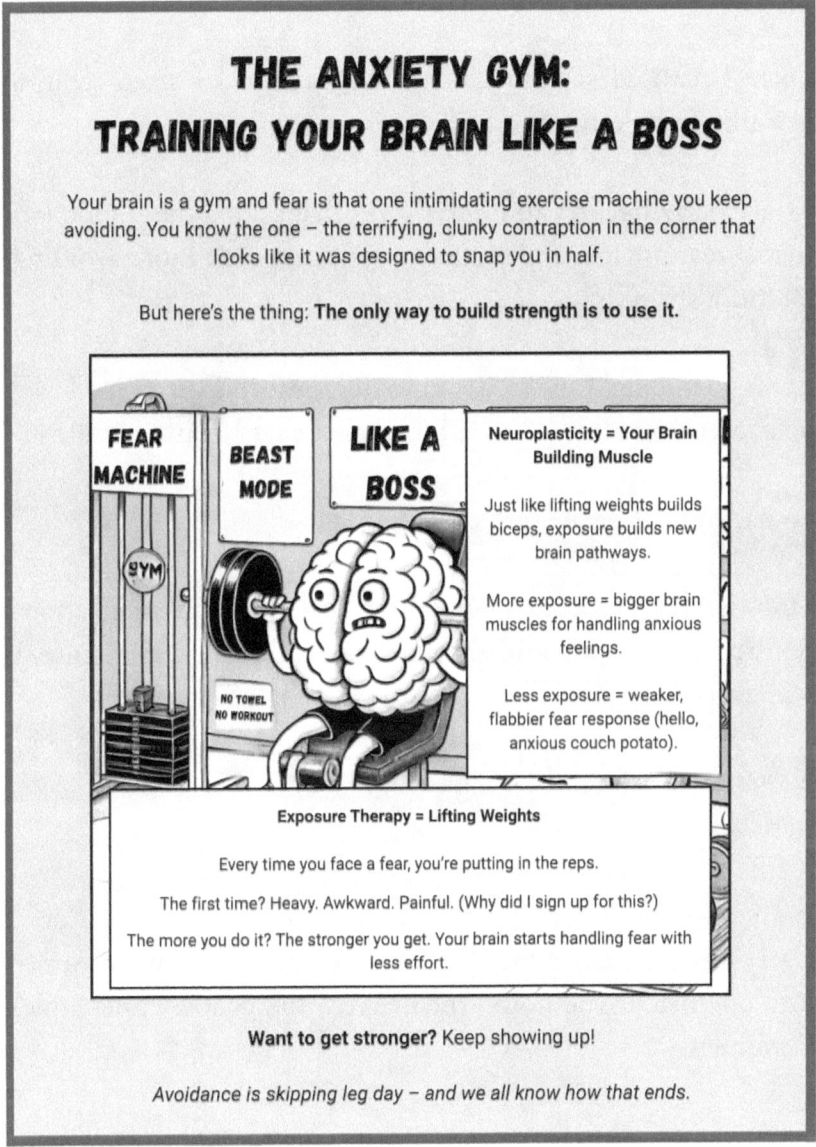

Of course, some fears are more than just 'reps at the gym' – deep-seated trauma or clinical anxiety might need extra support. But for everyday fears? Exposure works. And I unknowingly built my resilience one terrifying rep at a time.

From Theory to Action

Once I realised my brain could be trained, I started treating fear like a workout.

I started saying, *'Yes'* to more things that scared me. I took jobs that threw me into my biggest social fears – no more avoiding, no more shrinking.

Acting had taught me to step into discomfort. Every time I took on something scary, I proved to myself that I could handle it.

So naturally, I decided to up the ante.

I took a job that forced me into high-pressure social interactions, nonstop stimulation and absolutely no escape. It was intense. It was overwhelming.

It was bartending... In a nightclub.

A full-on sensory overload nightmare.

Everything I had spent my life avoiding was now crammed into one place: The noise, the crowds, the chaos. Panic attack imminent.

And yet... Nothing.

I was staying up until 2am, surrounded by the smell of beer and cigarettes, my ears buzzing from the bass.

Look at me go.

At first, I was just surviving. No safety net, no escape hatch – just me, a tray of drinks and a sea of strangers. Financial survival meant there was no choice but to push through. If I didn't work, I couldn't afford extras – clothes, entertainment. This money gave me a taste of freedom.

I didn't have a computer or the things other children had. My mum worked hard just to keep a roof on my head. She kept me grounded and I appreciate her every single day for that.

But looking back, I realise something now.

I wasn't just surviving – I was training my brain.

Every acting class, every nightclub shift, every terrifying public moment – I was rewriting the manual without even realising it.

And if I could do that by accident... What could I do on purpose?

The Fight I Didn't Need to Have

For what it's worth, anxiety has done a pretty solid job so far.

I mean, I'm still alive, right?

It's been my overprotective, slightly dramatic teacher since birth – throwing alarms, Screaming, *'DANGER!'* at everything from actual threats to mildly awkward conversations.

And honestly? It meant well.

At the time, I thought I was winning the battle against anxiety.

But I didn't realise yet – this wasn't a fight I was meant to win.

I wasn't supposed to defeat anxiety.

I was supposed to listen.

Anxiety wasn't a monster – it was a compass, pointing me toward the places that needed support. It was showing me where to look, where to heal and where I had been avoiding something important.

But I wasn't ready to trust it yet.

I still had my shield up, convinced I was in a battle I had to win.

And so, the fight continued.

ANXIETY CHEAT SHEET: What You Need to Know

Anxiety spent years convincing me it was a monster I had to defeat. Turns out, I had it all wrong.

Lesson 1: Confidence is Built Through Action (Not Before It)
Most people think confidence comes *before* you do the scary thing. Nope. It comes *from* doing.

TRY THIS: Instead of waiting to feel 'ready', pick one small thing outside your comfort zone and do it before you feel like you can. Your brain learns confidence by experience, not by waiting.

Lesson 2: Anxiety Isn't a Monster – It's A Map
Anxiety may be pointing toward the things you're avoiding, the places you need to grow and the work that needs to be done.

TRY THIS: Instead of asking, *'How do I get rid of this anxiety?'* try asking, *'What is this trying to show me?'* The answer might surprise you.

REMINDER: Confidence isn't something you wait for – it's something you build.

CHAPTER EIGHT

The Shape Shifter

"I became a mirror reflecting what everyone wanted to see, but somewhere along the way, I forgot my own reflection." (Sammy Barnett)

For years, confidence was my best mask – worn so often, I forgot what lay beneath.

I lived by the *'Be it until you see it'* motto, growing on the outside while slapping a plaster over something much deeper.

Up until my early 30s, I was a master of disguise – chameleon-like, always morphing into what others wanted. I was great at it. I could read a room like a script, blending in to survive.

But over time, survival turned into something else.

I had become a mirror, reflecting whatever each person wanted to see.

When I was with confident people, I became confident. When I was with those who struggled, I dulled myself down to match them. I couldn't be *too* confident – it wouldn't be relatable.

But the confidence mask always slipped. Because underneath – the insecurity, the fear, the need for approval – was still very much alive.

The Likeable Chameleon

I became incredibly likeable. Trusted by others. But deep down, I needed their approval.

And that, my friends, is where it gets messy.

I learnt early on that being easy-going and non-threatening was the surest way to be accepted. My nervous system *needed* that acceptance. On a primal level, being alone equalled danger.

Anxiety kept me in check.

Be likable. Stay in the tribe. Don't make waves.

But here's the kicker: People-pleasing often comes from a deep fear of rejection. It can feel like kindness, but at its core, it's about safety – the need to manage how others see us.

If I gave, gave and gave some more, I could *almost* control how people felt about me.

Spoiler Alert: You cannot control how people feel about you.

When I first heard that people-pleasing can be selfish, it stung. I thought I was being selfless and kind. But then I realised – it wasn't always about generosity. Sometimes it was about fear.

Fear of being disliked. Fear of making someone uncomfortable. Fear of rejection.

I wasn't just adapting to people – I was erasing myself.

The High Cost of People-Pleasing

People-pleasing is often a form of survival and tied to the brain's reward system. The problem? It's unsustainable. Constantly abandoning our own needs just to avoid a disappointed eyebrow raise?

Exhausting.

For me, even picking a restaurant for dinner felt as tense as defusing a bomb. The only casualty? My pride if someone hated the pasta.

I was like a walking *Pinterest* board – agreeable, but just a collection of borrowed opinions.

And when people noticed the contradictions, I felt exposed. I had spent so long shapeshifting, that I lost track of me.

I remember a friend discovering I loved classical music, despite acting like I was all about the heavy metal. *Korn,* eat your heart out! But my soul? It lit up for *Vivaldi Four Seasons* – a sound that echoed through my childhood home every Sunday.

I remember the stomach-dropping, blood-draining feeling of being confronted. It was awful. It might sound silly, but it felt very painful at the time.

For a long time, I internalised people's reactions – assuming I was the problem, when really, I was just their mirror.

But over the years, I have learnt something very powerful.

People's behaviours aren't them – they come out of fear or love. Fear of the unknown and impending death, or love for what they believe in.

And when you see it that way, compassion comes naturally.

Instead of trying to change people's perspectives, I recently started using Mel Robbins' *The Let Them Theory* (2023). (Big Mel fan here):

> ➤ Let them be afraid and judge the world around them.
> ➤ Let them live in fear of what could happen.
> ➤ Let me be open and get to know someone's story.
> ➤ Let me influence compassion, not fuel the fear inside others.

Understanding that so much of what people do is about survival – not malice – helped me soften my perspective. We adapt, we protect ourselves, we find ways to cope.

And just like I learnt to shape myself to meet expectations, I shaped my eating habits to meet my emotions – grabbing whatever was quick, easy and numbing.

Survival, in another form.

Eating my Feelings – and Paying the Price

You'd think, as a nutritionist, that food would've been front and centre.

It wasn't.

As a teenager, I found alcohol to be an easy way to relax at parties.

Drinking was socially acceptable, even expected.

For years, alcohol felt like my shortcut to confidence, my solution to social anxiety. But the next day? Anxiety came back – louder, sharper, more ruthless than before.

I wasn't just drinking for fun – I drank to quieten my nervous system.

But here's the thing: Alcohol doesn't actually turn down the volume. It just puts it on mute for a while. And when the effects wear off? The volume shoots back up – twice as loud.

I thought alcohol helped me escape anxiety, but in reality, it was feeding it.

The worst part? I didn't even realise I was stuck in the loop until much later.

It wasn't until I moved in with my husband (then boyfriend) that I really started noticing how food and alcohol made me feel. The sensitivities I had ignored for years finally caught up.

I hadn't studied nutrition yet, but I was connecting the dots.

Anxiety's lessons were still daily, but the tests weren't as constant. Some days were better, some were worse, but over time, I saw patterns. The more I listened to my body, the more I could work *with* it, instead of against it.

The stress of life still had a firm grip on my body and stress, as I would learn, hijacks everything – including food choices.

My husband was deep into fitness. Watching him inspired me. He meal prepped, weighed his food and talked about macros. The language of food, or so I thought.

At first, I just observed. Took mental notes.

I had already figured out that certain foods could trigger anxiety and panic. But knowing and doing? Two completely different things.

I *knew* sugar made me feel awful – jittery, panicked, exhausted. Yet every afternoon, like clockwork, I craved it.

It was my instant high, my temporary escape from the tension in my body.

Until one day, I hit a wall.

Mid crash, slumped on the couch, heart racing, hands shaking. My husband looked at me and said, '*You know, you don't have to feel like this.*'

It was such as simple statement, but it cracked something open inside me.

I didn't *have* to feel like this.

Maybe I had more control than I thought.

I had spent years believing my body and mind were at war – anxiety was just part of me, sugar cravings were just part of me. But what if they weren't? What if the choices I made could actually shift how I *felt*?

That was the beginning of something new – the first time I saw food as fuel, not just pleasure or punishment.

But breaking old habits wasn't just about knowing better – it was about rewiring my cravings, emotions and routines.

And sugar? It had me wrapped around its sticky little fingers.

Anxiety: The Best TEACHER You Never Asked For

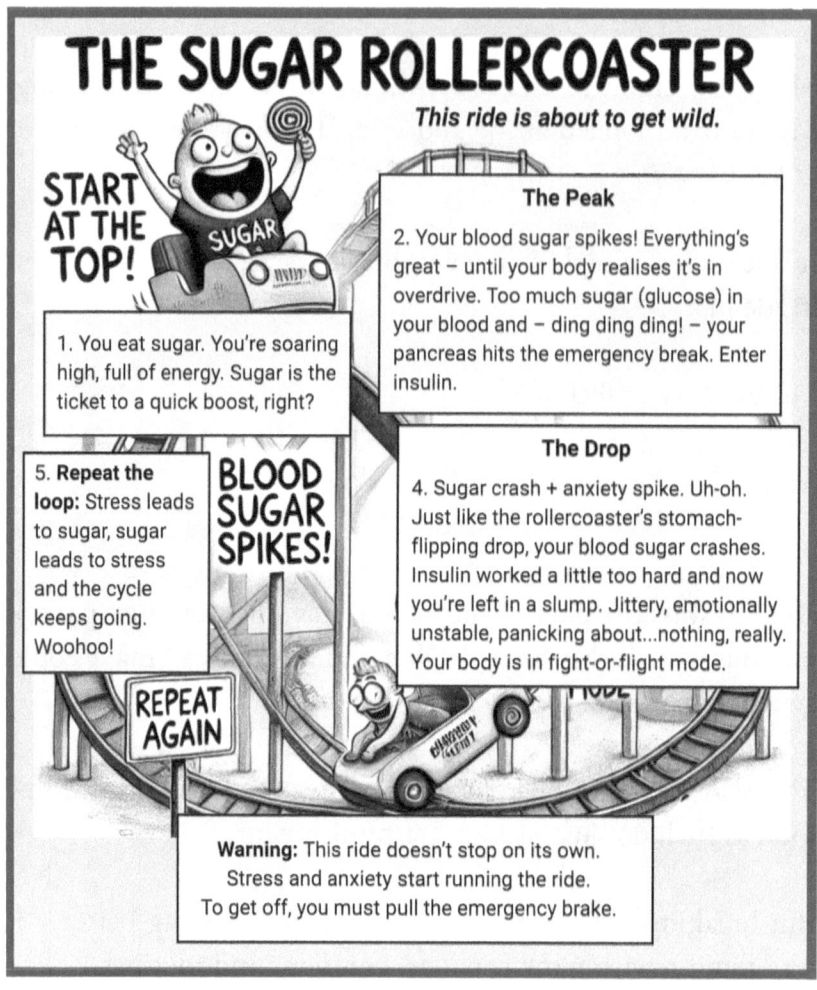

And it doesn't always start with sugar.

Back in primal times, when a tiger lurked in the bushes, your body knew exactly what to do – trigger the stress response and fuel up for the fight. And what's the quickest energy source? Glucose aka sugar.

Fast forward to today, there's no tigers. But your body doesn't know the difference. It's priming your muscles, flooding you with energy, gearing up for a sprint...except you're just sitting at your desk, stress-eating a *Krispy Kreme*.

Sugar wasn't the only thing keeping me stuck.

Alcohol was another sneaky passenger on this ride.

I had unknowingly trapped myself in a sugar-and-alcohol loop and my gut was paying the price.

Alcohol and sugar are the ultimate gut disruptors – the vodka-party-mixer dream team. My gut wasn't just struggling...it was explosive (pun intended).

For years, I ignored what my body was trying to tell me. Bloating, panic, fatigue – warnings I brushed off. But eventually, my body would force me to listen.

That's when I started noticing instead of numbing. And for the first time, my brain and body would feel stable.

But I wasn't there just yet.

Hello Movement, My Old Friend

When I moved more, I craved nutritious food. My body stopped screaming for sugar and started asking for nourishment. My brain felt clearer, more at peace.

Unlike food, exercise had always been my safe space.

As a child, I ran. I long jumped. Movement was built into my life – it was a given at school. I didn't have to think about it, plan for it, or make time for it. It was just there.

But once I left school, it wasn't automatic anymore.

Without structured sports or PE lessons, movement became something I had to actively choose. And for a while, I forgot how much I *loved* it.

Later, I found my way back – walking and cycling through the city, joining boot camps and now lifting weights. Not to *fix* myself, but because movement made me feel free. It made me laugh, smile and exhale.

And…for a moment…anxiety would take a personal leave day.

The Shape Shifter

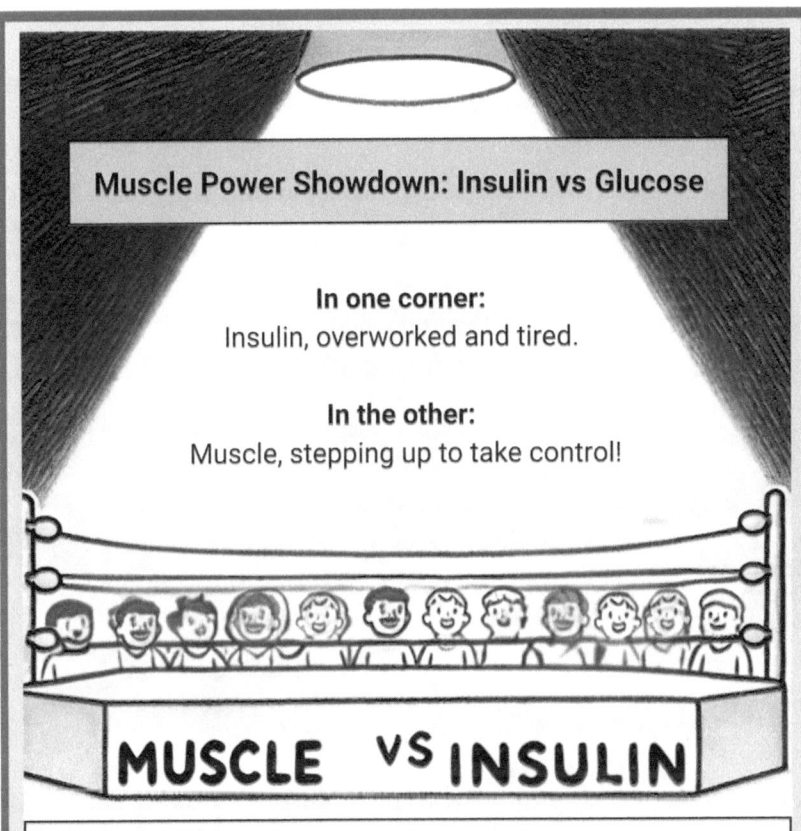

Muscle Power Showdown: Insulin vs Glucose

In one corner:
Insulin, overworked and tired.

In the other:
Muscle, stepping up to take control!

MUSCLE VS INSULIN

Round 1: Glucose Showdown
Muscle absorbs glucose like a sponge, keeping it out of the bloodstream. No more sugar chaos!

Round 2: Insulin Gets a Break
With more muscle, insulin can finally get some time off. Less sugar floating around means insulin doesn't have to work overtime.

Round 3: Anxiety Knockout
Muscle helps boosts mood and stability, kicking anxiety to the curb.

Winner: Muscle! Taking home the gold for better glucose control, less insulin strain and a huge anxiety win!

As I exercised more, I craved *nutritious* foods.

The 3pm sugar cravings? Gone.

My brain felt clearer, my energy steady. It was like I had found a reset button – not just physically, but mentally.

Nutrition and movement weren't just about health. They were about freedom. And I had found a partner who was just as invested in this journey as me.

And then something unexpected hit me…

Gratitude.

Gratitude Came Rolling In

Working in family and criminal law had given me a front-row seat to human suffering. I had been upgraded from receptionist to personal assistant, watching lives unravel before me.

And for the first time, I realised something that changed everything.

I was lucky. And I was grateful for it!

Yes, I had struggled. Yes, I had been trapped in anxious thoughts and spiralling emotions. But I had a mother who loved me. A sister who, despite our childhood fights, would always be there. A soon-to-be husband who wanted to build a safe life for us.

Even my little dog – my shadow through it all. Bless her little cotton socks.

Gratitude hit me like a tidal wave.

It wasn't just about appreciating what I had – it was about finally seeing my own worth beyond being a people-pleaser.

The more I nourished my body and mind, the more I started valuing myself outside of others' approval.

For so long, I lived like the star of my own drama series – victim, villain and maybe a touch of hero, but mostly stuck in the same sad loop.

I was alive, with people who loved me.

And then I saw it.

And it was about damn time.

My safe space was home. My soon-to-be husband became my rock – protective, steady, everything I needed.

But safety wasn't the same as growth.

And deep down, I knew I needed to start using my voice.

Finding My Voice

As I continued to grow, I realised I had to be more assertive – especially when it came to standing up for my future children. I had spent too long in passive or passive aggressive mode.

We've all played these roles, haven't we?

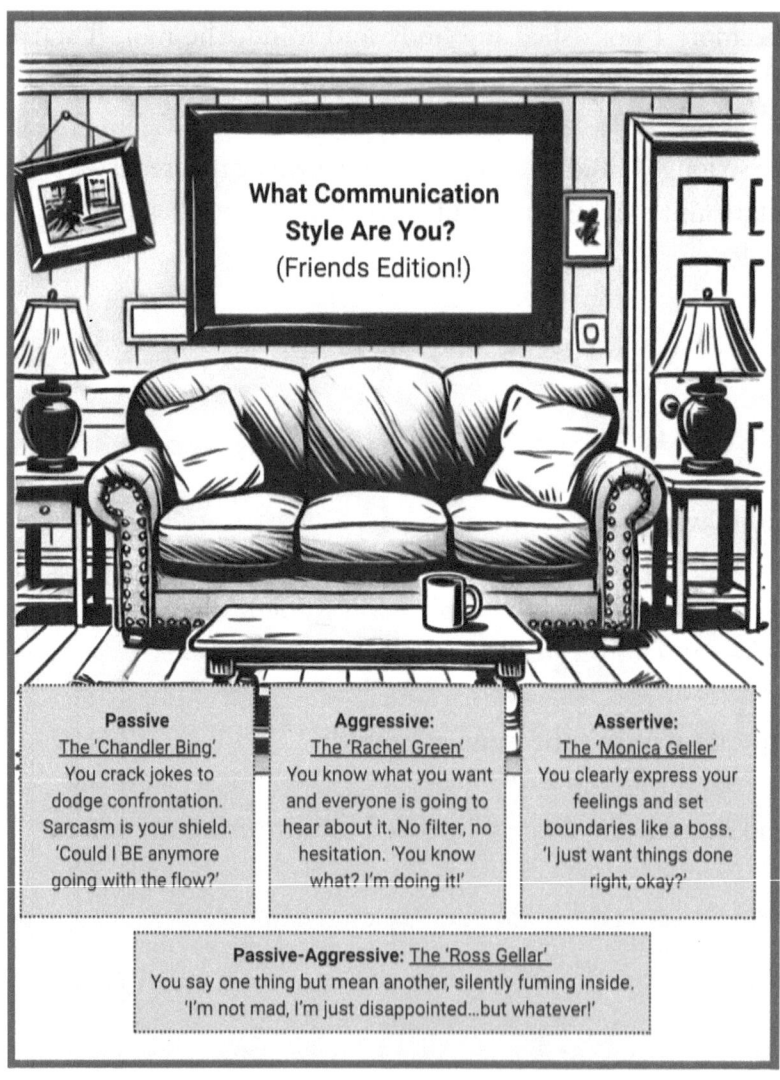

Of course, we're all a mix of different styles depending on the situation, but noticing these patterns can help you move towards a healthier, more assertive way of communicating.

Assertiveness didn't come naturally. I was Ross for a *very* long time. Telling everyone I was 'fine'.

Then I met my Monica. A friend who was unapologetically direct, asking for what she wanted without guilt, without over-explaining.

It was a revelation.

I couldn't keep adapting just to survive. I had to fight for myself and my future. But for all my social adaptability, there was one person I felt safe enough to practice with.

My husband.

Lucky him! I was about to practice speaking up – Monica style, but with a little less intensity.

At first, it was excruciating. My voice shook. My hands clenched. My stomach churned.

I had spent so long keeping the peace that saying what I needed felt…wrong. Like I was breaking some unspoken rule.

My husband, on the other hand?

He could say what he wanted without apologising, over-explaining, or second-guessing himself.

And that made me feel small.

Not because of him.

But because I didn't know how to do the same.

That's when I realised – this wasn't about a single conversation. This was about rewiring something deep inside me. I didn't just want to learn to be assertive.

I needed to.

For myself. For my family. For the life I was building.

But this shift wasn't easy. When we met, I was 17 and I was the Yes Girl. He was used to that version of me. When I started speaking up, setting boundaries, asking for what I needed – there was pushback. Not because he didn't love me, but because he had to see me in a new light.

And, honestly?

I was testing our relationship. Could this relationship shift into something I could grow in? One I could speak in? Be fully myself in?

I needed to know.

Because I wasn't going to stay the Yes Girl forever.

The Power of Vulnerability

Slowly, things changed.

I learnt that vulnerability – yes, vulnerability! – wasn't weakness. It was the thing that deepened my relationships, especially with my husband.

He saw I was trying. And as we communicated more, I finally learnt to express what I needed – not just as a wife, but as a mum, a woman and a human.

He may not speak the same emotional language as me, but he's learning.

And I'm learning, too.

Vulnerability isn't about oversharing or dumping emotions. It's about showing up as your full, messy, beautiful self and setting boundaries that serve you.

Even now, after almost 20 years of marriage, if I know what I want, I say it.

Clearly. Honestly. Even if it takes time (and maybe a few deep breaths).

Because it's important to stand firm, even when it's uncomfortable.

I used to think that being personable and likable meant I couldn't be assertive.

But that's just not true.

You can be both.

But being assertive wasn't just about speaking up in my personal life.

It extended into every part of who I was becoming – especially as I stepped into the world of business.

The Freedom of Boundaries

Boundaries – may be a harsh word for some, but for me?

It's survival. It's growth.

I learnt this even more when I started building businesses. Your time is precious. Say no to things that don't serve you. I continued to break free from external validation. And I realised: People-pleasing was just protection.

Thank you, anxiety, for those life lessons.

But now?

I got this.

The more you show up as the real you, whatever that looks like today, the less exhausting life becomes.

And, the best part?

The people who stick around?

They'll like you for *you*.

ANXIETY CHEAT SHEET: What You Need to Know

If you spend your life moulding to fit everyone else, you might forget who you are.

Lesson 1: People-Pleasing – Is it Kindness or Just Fear in Disguise?
People-pleasing isn't always selflessness – it can be self-abandonment.

TRY THIS: Next time you feel yourself saying *yes* out of guilt or obligation, pause and ask: *'Am I doing this out of love, or fear of disapproval?'* If it's fear, practice saying *'no'* – even just once. See how it feels.

Lesson 2: What You Eat (and Drink) Impacts More Than You Think
Sugar and alcohol can fuel anxiety, hormones, gut issues and emotional crashes.

TRY THIS: If your body is screaming at you, stop silencing it – start listening. Notice how certain foods make you feel. Jittery? Sluggish? Calm? Swap one thing this week – trade the afternoon sugar hit for something with protein and fat. See what happens.

Lesson 3: Assertiveness Isn't Aggression – It's Self-Respect
The right people won't leave because you say *no*.

TRY THIS: If setting boundaries feels impossible, start small:

Decide where to eat instead of saying, '*I don't mind!*' Express a preference, even if it feels uncomfortable.

The more you do it, the more you'll grow into the person you were meant to be.

REMINDER: The real you is always worth showing up for.

CHAPTER NINE

An A-type Awakening

"Anxiety and perfectionism are like dysfunctional besties – one fuels the other and together, they keep you in an exhausting loop." (Sammy Barnett)

I thought I could hold my world together by doing, achieving and controlling more. But the cracks were forming. I was too busy plastering over them with to-do lists and colour-coded schedules to notice.

The thing about anxiety? It doesn't always show up as panic and racing hearts. Sometimes, it has a clipboard, a stopwatch and a five-year plan. It whispers, *'Do more, be more, achieve more.'*

And before you know it, you're sprinting toward burnout, convinced that slowing down equals failure.

I thought being hyper-organised would keep anxiety in check. But the more I controlled, the more anxious I became.

It's like being behind the wheel of a car. Some of us floor it, some cruise and some over-plan every turn before we even start the engine.

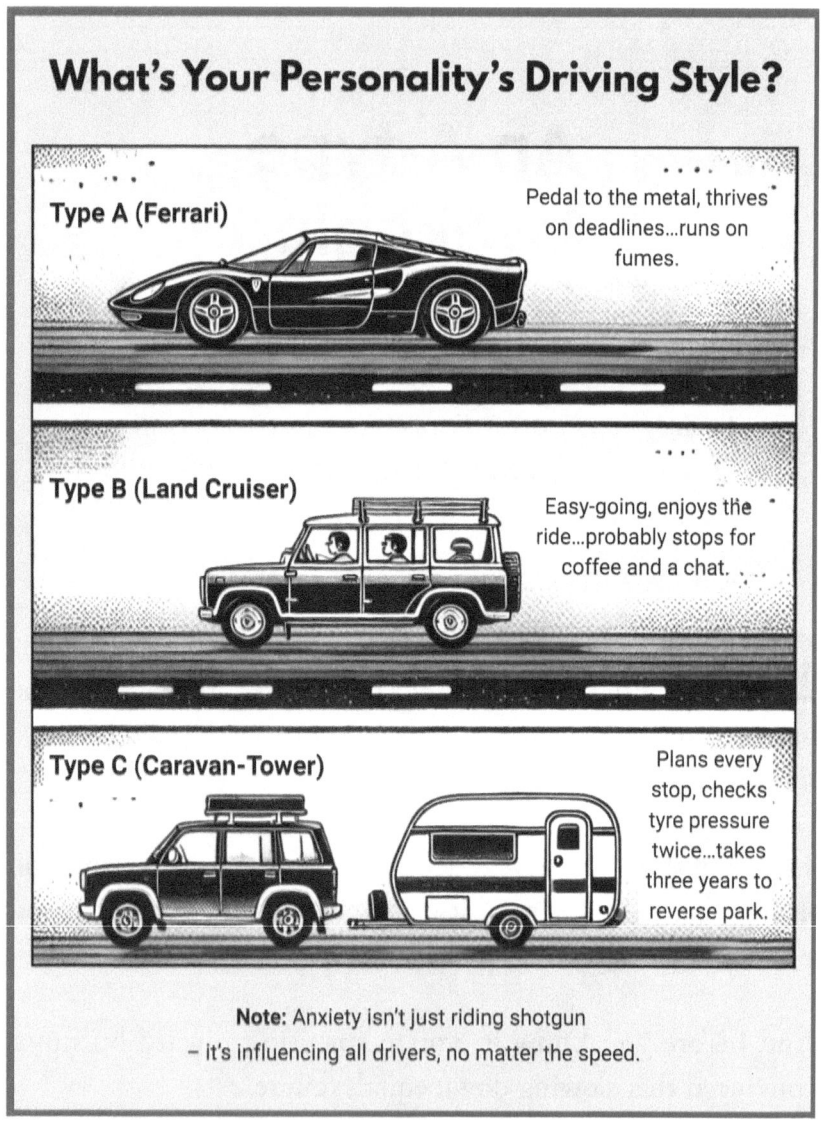

Hello, A-Type?

If you're a *Ferrari* like me, buckle up. Anxiety isn't just in the passenger seat – it's your backseat driver, barking instructions while you're too busy proving you can do it all.

Anxiety is like an exhausted teacher, sighing so hard she might pass out. *'Really? Another project? Haven't we been over this?'*

But you don't hear it. You're too busy juggling deadlines, running a marathon and checking off your to-do list every second. Anxiety's waving red flags, but you're too deep in hustle mode to notice. You're overloading yourself with work, double-booking your social life (if you still have one!) and telling yourself, *'No, I've got this!'*

Until you crash.

And anxiety? It's standing there, arms crossed. *Told ya!*

Anxiety gave you a list of things to do to feel safe. And you took it too far. Didn't you?! You did it all at once and had to learn the hard way (*again*).

People assume A-Types run on triple-shot lattes and energy drinks. Some of us – sure! But the truth? Many of us are caffeine-sensitive and need to put the cup down.

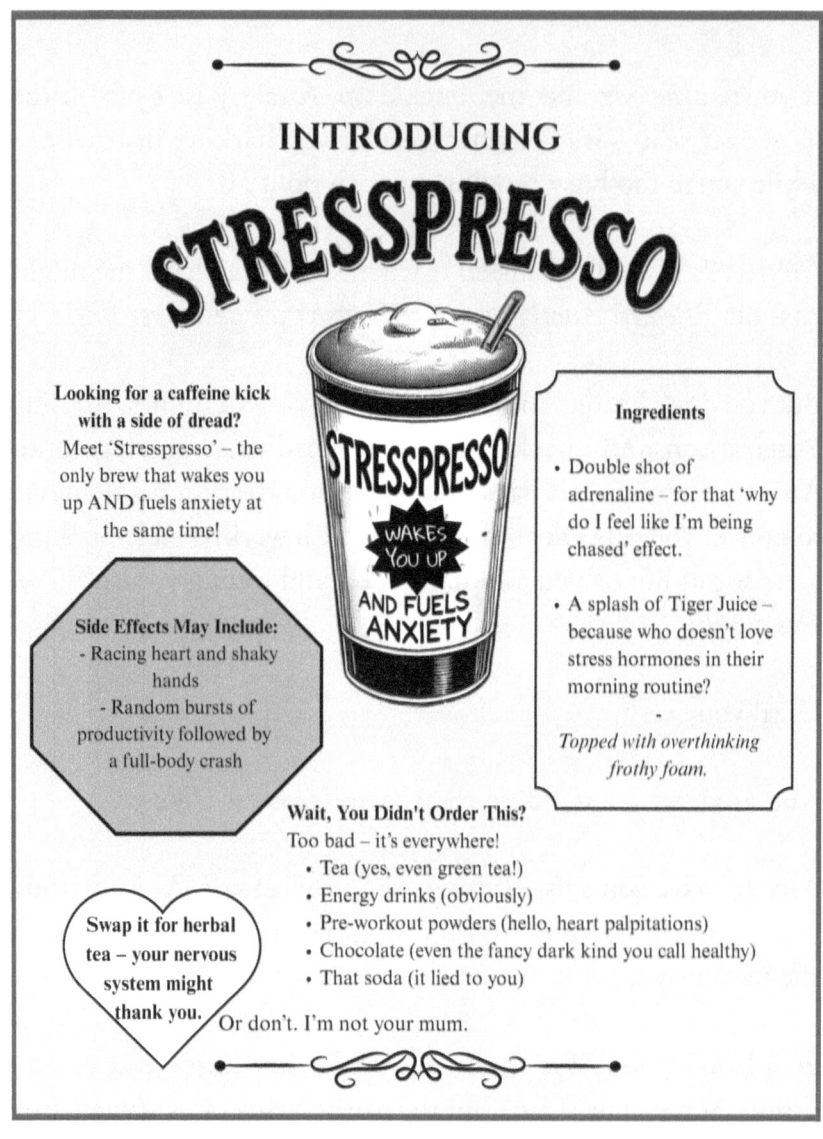

For many of us (especially those wired like a squirrel on *Red Bull*), caffeine can ramp up anxiety. But everyone's different – some can handle it, some can't.

My body does not need the extra buzz. It's already wired like someone who'd had five *Red Bulls*. Just ask my husband! *Twitch twitch.*

Same Patterns, Different Postcode

We moved to the suburbs – because that's where you're *'supposed'* to raise kids. Built a business, a house, a family. Two babies in. No sleep out.

Same patterns, different postcode. Now the 'Yes Mum', still overcommitted.

I became the go-to mum, always ready to help, always offering my time and energy to others. And I meant it – I genuinely wanted to be there. But looking back, I can see that sometimes, for my own health, I probably should have said *'no'*.

That being said, I *did* love hanging out with kids. Because, honestly? I still felt like one myself.

If you've ever seen me on stage at schools, you'd understand – I'm basically *Peter Pan* in female form.

The Invisible Weight We Carry

I was in full Mum mode – balancing nutrition, exercise, work and the illusion of control.

I looked like *Home Beautiful*. I lived like a hot mess.

I was nine months pregnant, running an online gift bag store in December (peak insanity), answering customer emails at midnight, literally working from my hospital bed while in labour.

When the contractions started…my first thought?

'I should finish packing today's orders.'

WHAT?!

Anxiety had me so deep in my 'must-do-it-all' mindset that I thought giving birth could wait. I was mentally exhausted, but my brain wouldn't let me stop. I wanted to prove I could do it all.

But to whom? I wasn't even sure anymore.

People praised me for it. *'Wow, you're amazing!'* And I ate it up. Meanwhile, I was one gust of wind away from plummeting. And behind the picture-perfect life?

The mental load of it all. What's that? The emotional burden we carry. It's like having 100 mental reminders open in your brain all at once.

Anxiety doesn't just give you tasks – it gives you an entire *mental symphony* of unfinished business playing on a loop.

'The Body Keeps the Score' (And Sends You the Bill)

Mothers do not get enough credit for the sheer mental load they carry.

All while:

- ➢ Growing humans
- ➢ Going through hormonal shifts
- ➢ Navigating relationships, careers and life
- ➢ And, as a fun bonus, triggering autoimmune diseases

Yes. AUTOIMMUNE DISEASES.

While there are many causes, stress can turn a slow burn into a wildfire.

I saw it in my clinic all the time – mums running themselves into the ground, their bodies breaking down under the weight of *doing it all*.

And still, they pushed through, convinced they could handle it.

Just like I did.

Until one day, I snapped.

I was standing in the kitchen, staring at the fridge, sobbing over a missing tub of yoghurt. At the time, I was running two businesses, pregnant, raising a toddler and keeping *everything* together – and yet, this damn yoghurt had me unravelling.

At the time, I didn't know if it was burnout, hormonal shifts, postnatal depletion – or all of the above. What I did know? That yoghurt wasn't the real problem. My nervous system had been running on fumes for too long.

My husband walked in, saw me crying and cautiously asked, *'Is this...about the yoghurt?'*

I wiped my tears and nodded.

'Yes. But also no. But mostly yes. But also life.'

And then, everything cracked. I'd gone from holding it together to screaming, shaking, completely unravelling.

Rage, panic, overwhelm. It all came rushing out in one uncontrollable wave.

And the worst part?

My baby felt it all. Every ounce of stress, fear, unravelling – he was absorbing it before he even took his first breath.

That still haunts me.

Anxiety wasn't even whispering anymore. It was screaming, throwing books, setting off alarms.

'You're breaking down... Stop!'

But I treated it like background noise, convinced I could power through. That's the thing about A-Types – we don't slow down until something forces us.

And something was about to force me.

The Storm Inside

I had no idea that inside my body, a silent storm was brewing.

My thyroid antibodies were rising, creeping toward what could be an autoimmune diagnosis I wouldn't see coming. Autoimmune diseases ran in my family, but I thought I was different.

I told myself I was fine. (I was not fine, but as mothers, we tell everyone we are.)

The truth is…

High-achieving women, especially mothers, are prime candidates for autoimmune issues. We're wired to push through, to carry the mental and emotional load, to put everyone else first. Chronic stress doesn't just make us tired – it rewires our entire system. Over time, high levels of Tiger Juice can weaken our immune system. It can open us up to inflammation and autoimmunity.

Stress messes with our hormones too which play a role in our immune function.

Wild fact. About 80% of all autoimmune conditions occur in women (Ngo et al., 2014). They can flare up during major hormonal shifts like:

- ➢ Pregnancy
- ➢ Postpartum
- ➢ Perimenopause

While the exact link isn't fully understood, the connection between stress, hormones and immunity is undeniable.

Being a woman is grand.

I thought I was proving my strength – keeping it all together. But the truth?

I was falling apart. And my body was paying the price.

Anxiety fuels the fire. Stress sparks inflammation, and inflammation feeds anxiety.

And honestly? We've been set up for this – by society, by expectations, by the belief that slowing down or pausing is failing.

I didn't see it then, but looking back, anxiety was waving every red flag possible. I just wasn't slowing down long enough to notice.

Sprinting Toward Burnout

Every time someone told me, '*You need to rest*,' I'd nod politely and then immediately add five more things to my to-do list. Slowing down felt *dangerous*.

What if I stopped achieving and lost my identity?

What if I wasn't *needed* anymore?

What if I had to sit with my own thoughts and realise…I wasn't okay?

Rest wasn't a break – it was a threat.

So, I kept sprinting, ignoring the fact that I was heading straight toward burnout at *Ferrari* speed. And when you live life in the fast lane, you don't just juggle responsibilities – you perfect them.

The Cost of Perfection

I wasn't just a high-achiever. I was a high-achiever with a clipboard, a colour-coded planner and a desperate need for control.

- Perfect schedules
- Perfect home
- Perfect Mum

I was determined to do it all.

One moment, I was on top of the world – checking off lists, meal-prepping like a pro, managing life like a well-oiled machine.

The next?

I was crying in the shower, screaming in my car, raging at nothing and everything. I didn't want my children to see me like that. So, I did what any good perfectionist would do – I built more systems to keep the chaos under control.

So. Many. Systems.

At first, it worked.

Until it didn't.

Because eventually, I wasn't running my life. My systems were. They were overcomplicated, overloaded with last-minute changes and somehow, despite all the planning, no one actually knew what was going on except me.

I was drowning in my own efficiency.

I couldn't function without a checklist. I couldn't rest without guilt.

I couldn't stop.

Even when I was exhausted. Even when I was falling apart.

Because in my mind, slowing down meant failing. And that couldn't happen. Perfectionism wasn't just a personality quirk.

It was my defence mechanism. A way to control the chaos. A way to keep anxiety quiet.

I told myself:

'If I get everything right… If I never drop the ball… Maybe I'll never feel this gnawing fear.'

But anxiety isn't silenced by perfectionism. If anything, she feeds on it. And I was feeding her well. I was running myself into the ground, but I wasn't about to stop.

Not yet.

Because stopping meant facing the thing I'd been avoiding all along.

Super Mum Syndrome

Let's be real – social media has us all believing that motherhood looks like themed lunchboxes and colour-coordinated playrooms.

The truth? Even the most picture-perfect mum's have chaos behind the scenes. I know this because I was one of them.

Maybe not to that extent – but parts of me were there.

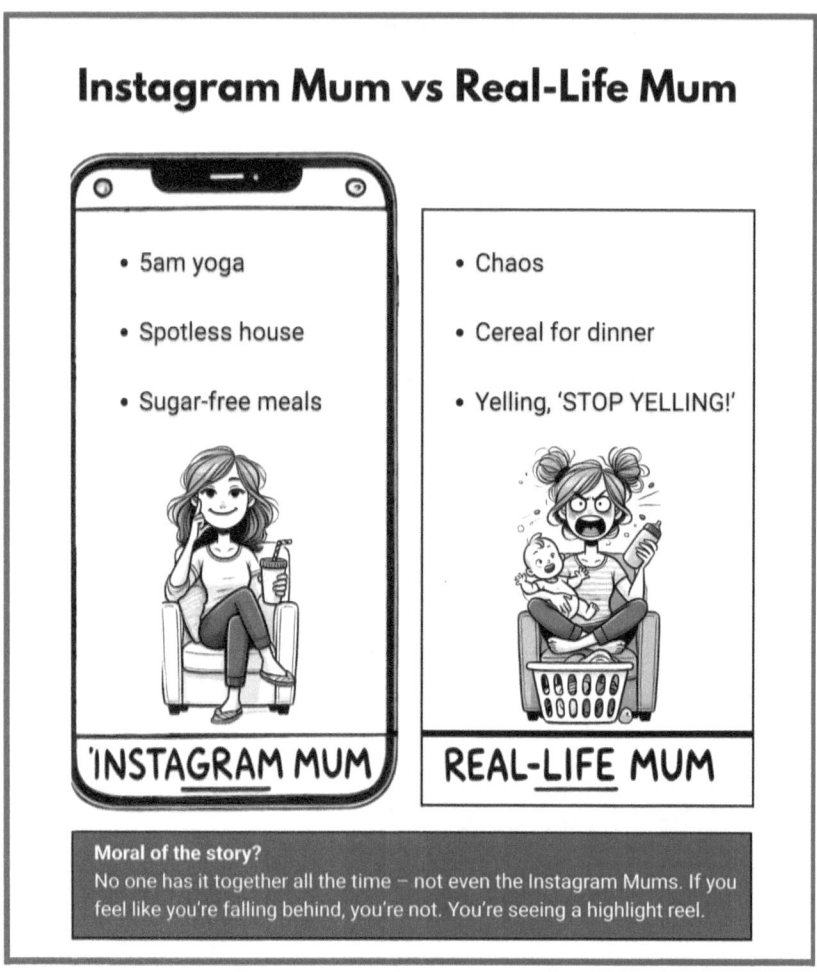

Pick your battles, ditch the guilt. Some women genuinely enjoy doing all this, we don't have to follow suit. We get to prioritise. We get to pick and choose what matters.

And the fact that we even *worry* about being a 'bad' mum? That means we are *'great'* mums. If we truly didn't care, we wouldn't even question it…

Your mental health matters more than a *Pinterest*-worthy bento box. Mothers are overworked, overwhelmed and constantly on the verge of burnout. It's time we start showing each other the truth of it all. And stop tearing each other down – as mothers and in business.

But at the end of the day, the pressure isn't just coming from social media. Sometimes, our harshest critic isn't an influencer with a perfectly curated feed. It's that other voice inside our head.

The one named 'mum guilt'.

The Gut-Punch Moment

Mum guilt is brutal.

Despite my own struggles back then, I loved my children fiercely. They were (and still are) my greatest joy and so much of my gratitude is for them. No matter how lost I felt inside, I poured everything I had into giving them a life filled with fun, adventure and love. Because if nothing else, I wanted them to know happiness was possible.

And maybe – just maybe – there was a hint of mum guilt lurking beneath it all, nudging me to overcompensate, to be everything, to make up for the moments when I wasn't fully present.

One day, my son came home with a Mother's Day questionnaire from school. It asked:

'What's your mum's favourite thing to say?'

And in his tiny, adorable handwriting, he wrote, '*In a minute.*'

I stared at that paper for so long.

It hit me like a punch to the gut – he wasn't hearing '*I love you*' or '*I'm so proud of you.*' He was hearing '*In a minute*' because I was always rushing, always ticking things off a never-ending list.

That moment wrecked me. Because I realised…

My to-do list was parenting my kids more than I was. I was so busy trying to '*do it all*' that I forgot to show them it's okay **not** to.

That it's okay to be messy.

That it's okay to be human.

That it's okay to cry when life gets hard.

But instead of letting his words pull me under, I let them wake me up. Sometimes, it's the smallest shifts – pausing to listen, saying yes to what matters – that change everything.

Because life can be tough.

The world can be tough.

And mum guilt knows exactly where to hit you.

She whispers:

An A-type Awakening

'You could be doing more.'
'You should do better.'
'You're failing.'

But I learnt – slowly and painfully – that kids don't need a perfect mum. They need a present mum.

A mum who lets go.

A mum who laughs more than she stress-cleans.

A mum who knows that a banana for dinner is acceptable sometimes.

I had to reconnect with my body and give it what it actually needed. And letting go?

It was the hardest thing I'd ever have to do.

But I wasn't ready to give it all up yet. I was holding onto perfectionism so tightly, convinced that if I just:

- Did more
- Organised more
- Achieved more

…maybe I could finally quieten the guilt.

But the harder I tried, the worse it got. Because this wasn't just about being a *'good mum'* – it was about *me*. And my own impossible standards. About never feeling like I was enough. And that's when the identity crisis hit.

When Success Still Feels Like Failure

Post-natal depression came on thick.

Super Mum Syndrome was me trying to do it all. But postnatal depression? That was a whole different beast. I thought I just wasn't coping, but looking back, I can see it was more than that.

I felt like I had lost an identity that, if I'm honest, I probably never really had in the first place. I was a stay-at-home mum, trying to build something of my own.

Meanwhile, my husband's business was growing.

At this stage of life, that's all it felt like. His business. His success. He was the one bringing in the money while I sat at home, working a few days a week, trying to prove that I could do it, too.

Ridiculous. Right?

Talk about a high-achieving woman who was never good enough in her own mind. I built our family business with him, but I didn't see it that way.

In my eyes… I was a failure.

So, I kept setting impossibly high expectations. I kept striving for perfection in every way. Because for years, I thought my worth was in:

- How much I could achieve
- How perfect I could make everything

But anxiety had been trying to tell me to slow down all along. Life isn't about proving my worth through achievements. It's about being present. Being real.

And sometimes?

Just being.

And maybe, just maybe – that was the A-Type awakening I needed all along.

ANXIETY CHEAT SHEET:
What You Need to Know

If you think perfectionism is just a personality trait, think again – it's often anxiety in disguise.

Lesson 1: Perfectionism Isn't Productivity – It's a Fear Response
Colour-coded schedules may help ease anxiety but shouldn't become a coping mechanism for avoiding discomfort.

TRY THIS: Next time you find yourself fixating on getting everything 'just right', ask:

'Am I organising to support myself, or to avoid feeling anxious?'

If it's the latter, challenge yourself to leave one thing imperfect. *Yes, on purpose. Imprefectly.*

Lesson 2: Is Your To-Do List Raising Your Kids
The mental load of motherhood is real, but kids don't need a perfect mum – they need a present one.

TRY THIS: Pick one daily moment to slow down and be fully present. Sit down at the dinner table instead of multitasking. Pause and actually listen when they tell you a story. Say 'yes' to a moment of connection instead of 'in a minute.'

Lesson 3: Slowing Down Feels Like a Threat – But It's Actually the Cure

Burnout doesn't prove your strength – it proves you're human.

TRY THIS: Schedule one guilt-free, totally unproductive hour this week.

No work. No chores. No justifying why you *deserve* the break.

Notice the discomfort. That's your conditioning talking – not reality.

REMINDER: Your worth isn't in how much you do. Now, take a breath. *For real this time!*

CHAPTER TEN

Eating My Way to Immortality

*"What you eat matters.
But so does what you think, say and do.
That's where real health begins."* (Sammy Barnett)

Motherhood and moving home had swallowed my routines whole. My carefully structured health habits? Vanished. Meal prepping? A distant memory. Life had become messy and unpredictable. But I knew nutrition and fitness weren't just about looking good – they were my anchors.

Without them, I felt lost. It was time to bring them back!

I dove into my studies – not just for my family, but me. I needed something beyond motherhood, something that reminded me who I was before the chaos. Being a mum was one of my greatest joys, and I know for many women it's the destination they dreamt of. But I couldn't shake the sense that I was meant to explore more – not instead of motherhood, but alongside it.

So, I signed up for a life-changing four-year course to become a clinical nutritionist. No idea how I'd fit that in, but it was something just for me. And of course, I felt guilty about that, too.

Anxiety had always been my unwanted sidekick, whispering worst-case scenarios. In the past, it had gripped me through panic attacks and avoidance. But now? It had found a new playground – nutrition. If I could just control what went into my body, maybe I could control how I felt.

Maybe I could even outrun fear itself.

Unlocking the Body's Secrets

What started as a way to reclaim my identity quickly became something more. I wasn't just studying nutrition – I was decoding every symptom I'd ever had.

For years, I had searched and stayed up late chasing answers. The human body wasn't just functional – it was extraordinary.

And now? I had the blueprint.

I had the knowledge to heal myself, protect the people I loved and run a clinic to help others do the same. Anxiety had always made me feel powerless, but this? This gave me control. If I could decode how my body worked, maybe I could finally outmanoeuvre anxiety rather than be its victim.

Looking back, I see it clearly – anxiety had been guiding me all along, nudging me toward answers I didn't even know I was looking for. While I was studying the body to understand life, deep down, I was doing it to avoid…death.

But while I was mapping out the body's blueprint, one system in particular kept demanding my attention – my gut. No matter how much I learnt, digestion remained a daily battle. It was time to put my knowledge to the test.

Trust Your Gut

For years, my gut was a full-blown rebel. Bloating, IBS, mad dashes to the toilet (TMI I know, but let's be real). You're wondering what TMI means now? Aren't you? My gut and brain were basically in a toxic relationship (it's 'Too Much Information' if you were still wondering and hadn't Googled it yet).

My gut issues weren't just physical – they were part of a pattern. Anxiety had always made me hyper-aware, always questioning, always investigating. Now, that same relentless curiosity was driving me to figure out my own biology.

I learnt I had SIBO – Small Intestinal Bacterial Overgrowth. Bacteria had set up camp where it shouldn't, fermenting my food and leaving me feeling like a balloon animal after every meal. It wasn't just bloating me up. It was also triggering things inside me that made me feel even more on edge.

If I wanted to heal, I thought I had to start here.

Anxiety: The Best TEACHER You Never Asked For

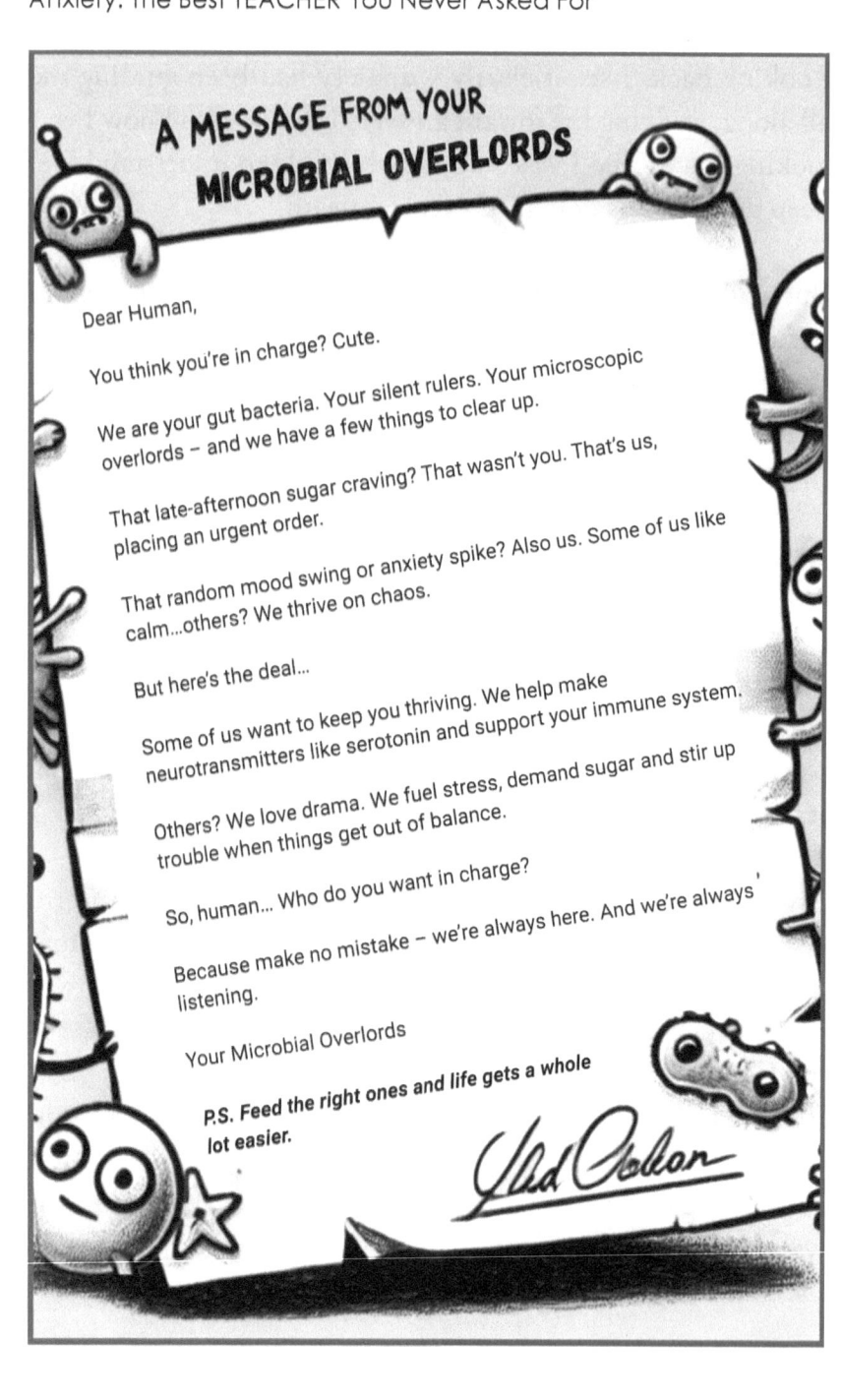

Gut bacteria 'chat' with the brain, influencing mood and anxiety. After reading *The Psychobiotic Revolution* (2017), it made me realise I wasn't just dealing with gut issues – I was biologically outnumbered. 10 bacterial cells for every human one. Other studies show it may actually be closer to one to one (Sender et al., 2016). Phew!

So…was I actually in charge? Or were my gut bacteria cosplaying as me?

These gut imbalances weren't just messing with my digestion – they were messing with my mind. Some gut bacteria cranked up anxiety, while others sent out chill signals.

Research is still unfolding, but one thing became clear – my microbes were messing with my mood.

Knowing this was one thing but fixing the problem was another. If I wanted to feel better, I had to go beyond just knowing. I had to rebuild my gut from the inside out.

Laying the Groundwork for a Happy Gut

Rebalancing my gut wasn't just about adding good bacteria – I had to make a home where they could thrive. Years of stress and imbalance had left my digestive tract like dry, cracked soil. Before I could grow the good guys, I had to repair the damage.

I repaired my gut with things like slippery elm, glutamine, zinc and bone broths. Ceylon cinnamon and chromium curbed sugar cravings – less sugar, fewer bad bacteria tantrums. This was my path, not a universal prescription. Everyone's gut has different needs. And before you go out and buy these things (because that's what I would've done), I encourage you to keep reading this book.

Once my gut wasn't under attack 24/7, the good guys could thrive.

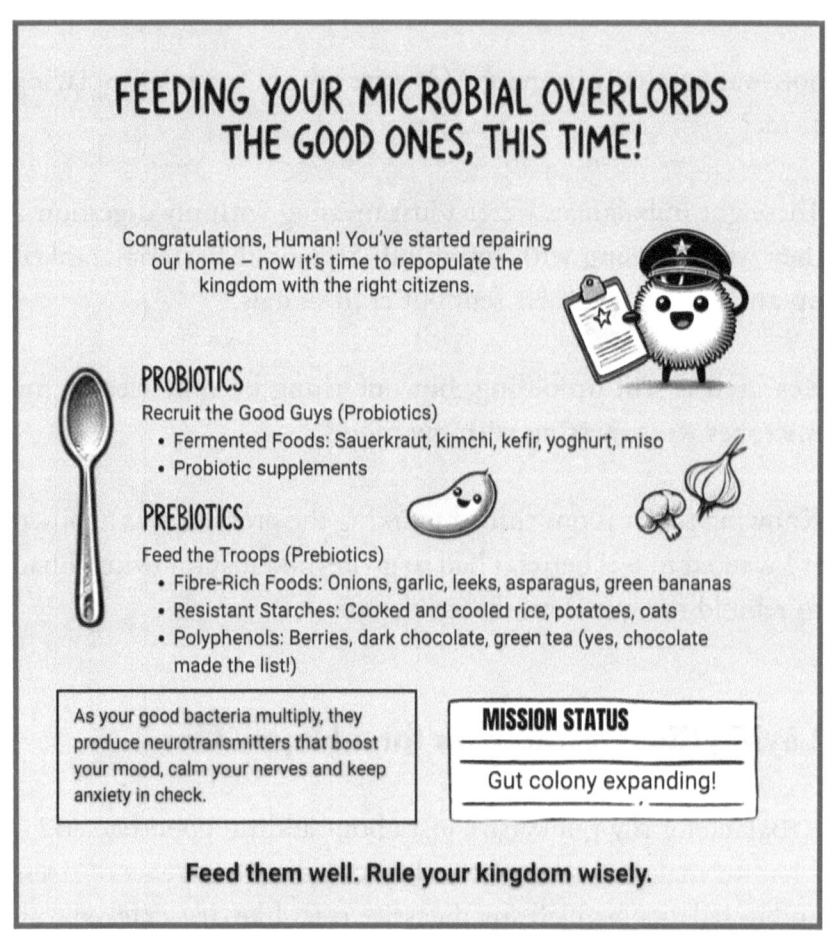

As I dug deeper, I started uncovering common food sensitivities – gluten, dairy…the usual suspects. At the time, these foods seemed to be triggering gut issues and aggravating anxiety. So, I ditched them.

But then? I went full nutrition detective. If the soil was depleted of nutrients, so was my plate. I wasn't settling for food stripped of its nutrients. I wanted the real stuff – straight from the good soil and most definitely not a lab.

Sounds like the perfect plan, right? Cut out problem foods, flood my gut with good bacteria, load up on fibre and whole foods and *boom!*

- Better digestion
- Better mood
- Better life

And for some people, that's exactly how it plays out.

But here's what I was about to learn the hard way – nutrition isn't a one-size-fits-all formula. What heals one person, can backfire on another. And sometimes? Too much of a good thing becomes the problem.

Rebalancing my gut was a game-changer, but anxiety still had its claws in me. That's when I stumbled upon another major player in the anxiety puzzle – neurotransmitters.

Boosting My Neurotransmitters

I had learnt that dopamine and serotonin were largely made in the gut. But now I discovered another key player: GABA – the ultimate calm-down neurotransmitter. Without enough GABA, anxiety runs wild.

Another key to boosting these chemical messengers? Protein.

Without this, my body couldn't make enough neurotransmitters.

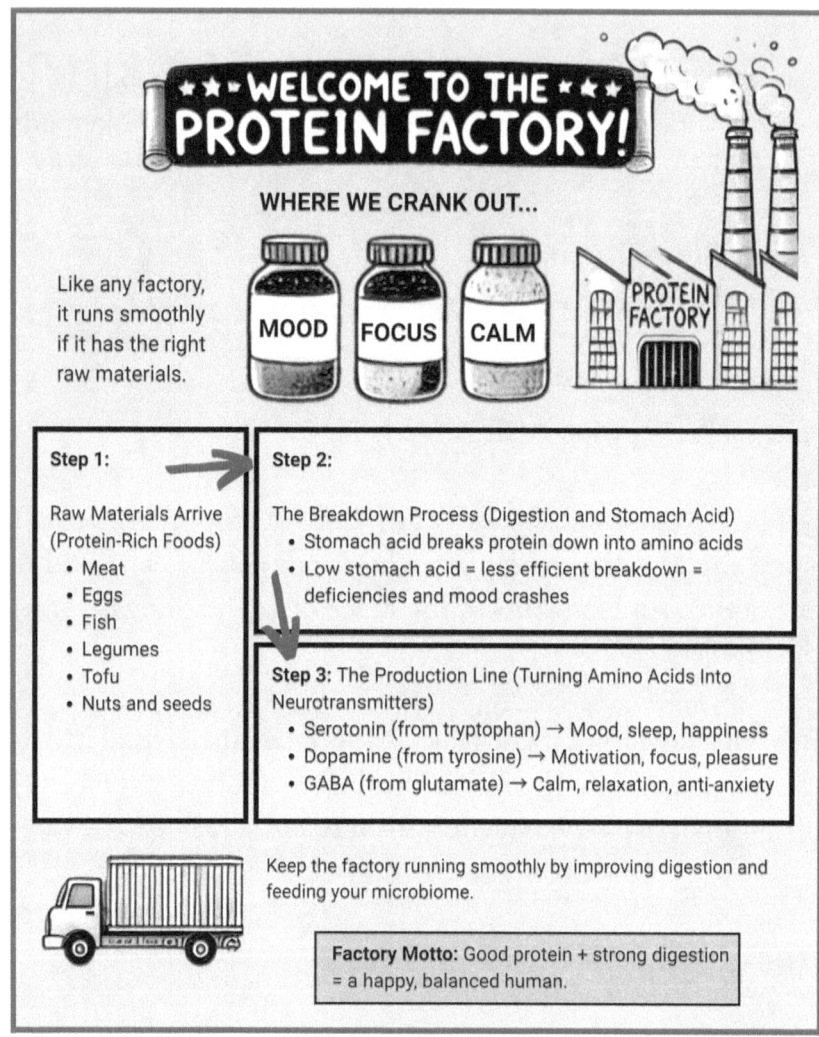

Without a good source of protein, our bodies may struggle to produce enough serotonin (hello, mood boost!) or dopamine (hello, motivation!). Protein quickly became my new best friend.

A strong, healthy gut brings in good bacteria and helps breakdown protein into amino acids – the very building blocks of neurotransmitters that keep me balanced. Got it!

But it wasn't just about making neurotransmitters – I needed to know if my body had the raw materials to produce them in the first place. That meant diving deeper into nutritional testing to uncover what was missing.

Because while amino acids might be the building blocks, vitamins and minerals are the architects – directing each step, ensuring those blocks converted into the neurotransmitters my body needed to function. Without them? The whole structure crumbles.

Running on Empty

My gut was healing, my neurotransmitters were firing but something still felt off.

I had spent my life sensing imbalance, like I was always one step away from an answer. Now, I had tools to stop guessing and start testing. Maybe anxiety had trained me for this – to see connections where others didn't, to question everything, to chase solutions others overlooked.

Nutrients weren't just fuel; they were essential workers in the biochemical pathways that kept my brain and body running. Without the right ones, no amount of gut healing or neurotransmitter boosting would be enough.

So, I dove into blood testing for key nutrients that impact mental health.

And what I found? I was running on empty.

Chronic stress had burned through my most important nutrients – fast. I was in deficit mode.

Stress depletes:

> - Magnesium – Our nervous system's chill pill
> - B Vitamins – Brain fuel and energy (without them, mood and focus tank)
> - Zinc – Essential for stress resilience and gut repair

And to top it off? My Vitamin D was very low. This is crucial for serotonin and immune function. And without enough magnesium, my body couldn't even activate it from the sun.

I wasn't just *low* in nutrients – I was running a biochemical debt.

Biochemically bullied and in debt.

No wonder I felt drained.

This was another wake-up call. Mental health wasn't just about mindset. It was chemistry. And if I wanted to feel better, I needed to replenish what stress had stolen.

Eating My Way to Immortality

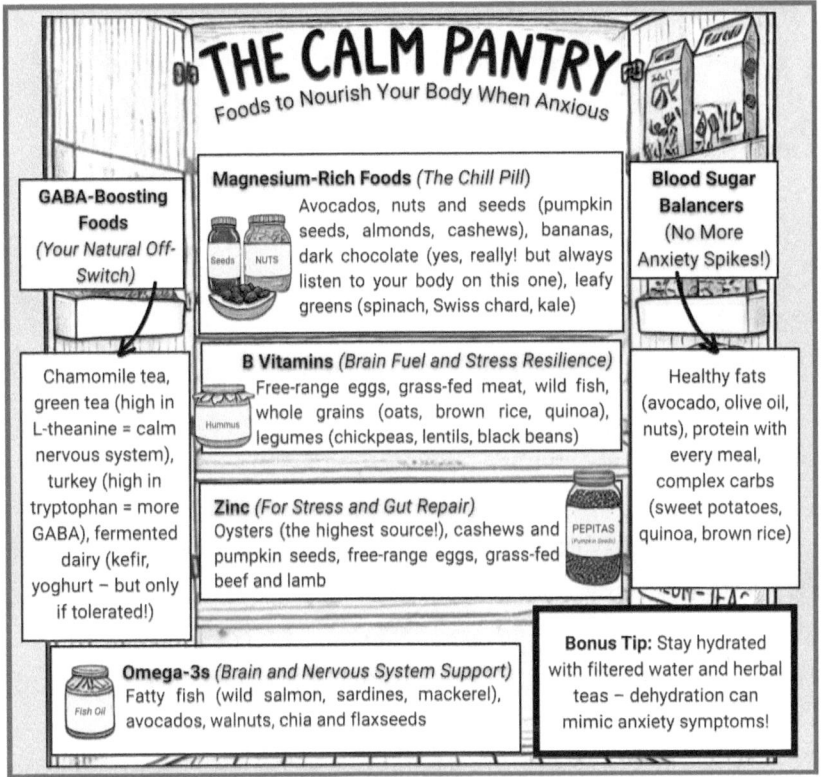

At first, I believed food could fix *everything*. But then I discovered something even more powerful.

Biohacking My Brain (and Why it Backfired)

I experimented with neurotransmitter precursors, convinced I could bio-hack my way to feeling amazing.

L-tryptophan for serotonin, L-tyrosine for dopamine, GABA for instant chill.

Of course, there are other neurotransmitters and amino acids (just like with vitamins, minerals and other key nutrients), but if I mentioned them all, this book would be about 1,000 pages longer.

For a while, I was biohacking like a pro – better sleep, sharper focus, more control.

Until I realised…I was playing Jenga with my body's chemistry.

Supplements – especially those affecting neurotransmitters – can be just as risky as medication. The wrong form or dose can throw everything off balance. That's why working with a professional is key.

Instead of fixing anxiety, I was fuelling it. It was not happy.

What started as a 'shortcut to balance' become yet another lesson in how too much control can backfire.

What I learnt (the hard way):

- Nutrients work together – you can't always isolate one and expect miracles.
- Not all supplements are created equal – form and absorption matter.
- Deficiencies can keep anxiety cycles going, but more of a particular nutrient isn't always the answer.
- Testing gave me real answers, but even then…*more wasn't always better.*

The more I learnt, the more I realised mental health wasn't a one-and-done fix – it was a biochemical puzzle. And puzzles? I love puzzles!

I couldn't wait to open my clinic and help people solve theirs.

But just when I thought I had all the pieces… things were about to get messy.

What had started as healing, had become an obsession.

When 'Healthy' Eating Becomes A Prison

At first, I thought I was healing. But looking back, I see anxiety had just shape-shifted. Where it once made me fear the outside world, now it made me fear food.

Same detective brain – just a new case to solve.

I became obsessed with 'clean eating'. Everything had to be organic. I became fixated on cutting out sugar. I consumed endless articles linking sugar to anxiety, mood swings and even disease – each one reinforcing my fear.

I did all the diets – Paleo, Keto, vegan, gluten free, dairy free… you name it.

I was taking so many supplements… I rattled when I walked.

This extended to my children. They weren't allowed certain foods. My mum was too scared to feed them anything when she babysat. My son called milk 'cow's milk', like it was some foreign delicacy.

When I graduated, I was testing everything – blood, poop, urine, saliva, hair. I fell into the trap of believing that perfect health meant ultimate control over my body.

I wanted my children to be healthy, but I didn't realise my rigid approach was creating fear around food. Perfection became the goal – and the cost? My sanity. My energy. My sleep. I was running on Tiger Juice and willpower, convinced that if I just controlled one more thing, I'd finally feel safe.

I thought I was winning, but I was just feeding my fear.

The *Jenga* tower was wobbling.

Anxiety screaming, *'STOP!'* It had given me the manual to keep me safe around foods and toxins and I took it to the next level.

I didn't listen.

This obsession led me into Orthorexia – an extreme fear of *'unhealthy'* foods. I spent hours analysing every ingredient, refusing to eat unless it was 'clean'. I became fixated on toxins, convinced anything less than *perfect* was harmful.

It wasn't until later I realised how far I'd gone. And I wasn't alone. Many nutritionists and health professionals walk a fine line between education and obsession and I unknowingly crossed it.

Burnout from extreme dietary control is real. Studies show that rigid eating patterns and food fear can actually increase anxiety rather than reduce it (Strahler & Stark, 2023).

But at the time? I thought I was hacking the system.

I thought I was getting healthier, but really, I was getting stricter. More rules, more restrictions, more control. And like every time I'd tried to control anxiety before – it was about to backfire.

The Calm Before the Storm

Then, because clearly I hadn't pushed myself far enough, I decided to enter a fitness competition. Slashing calories while training every day? Genius move.

My body had tried subtle hints. Then urgent nudges. Then a full-blown alarm system. Anxiety was the teacher and I was failing. Hard. Time to pay attention. Or not…

In school, anxiety made me avoid everything. Now, it made me do the opposite – hyper-focus, over-control, chase perfection. Same anxiety, different disguise. And just like before, I was about to learn the hard way that control is not the same as peace.

I threw myself into the intense training, obsessive meal prep, micromanaging everything. I had never been one to count or restrict calories, but now? I was doing all of it. Weighing every meal, avoiding anything remotely 'toxic', convinced that discipline was the key to proving my worth – and maybe even make me immortal.

And for a while? It worked.

I felt like the old 'pre-panic' me. I felt stronger, sharper, confident. The girl I thought I'd lost forever.

I found her again!

I felt unstoppable. The *'Believe it until you see it'* attitude that propelled me through life? It was back, living inside me.

But… There's *always* a but.

I had pushed myself beyond what was healthy.

And soon, my body would scream so loudly, I would *have* to listen.

Anxiety wasn't something to defeat – it was something to be understood. For years, I thought health was the answer to anxiety. But really, anxiety had led me to understand health.

My gut, my brain, my body – none of them were the enemy. They were just trying to tell me something.

And the more I listened, the more I realised that true health isn't about control.

It's about trust.

Trusting my body. Trusting that I don't have to micromanage every bite to feel safe.

ANXIETY CHEAT SHEET: What You Need to Know

Health isn't about perfection and control isn't the same as safety.

Lesson 1: Your Gut is the Loudest Student in Class
Ignore your gut long enough and it'll start throwing tantrums.

TRY THIS: Consider feeding the good bacteria (they literally control your mood). This week, try adding a probiotic food, a prebiotic food or a little more fibre. Working with a professional is important to track changes and notice what makes things better (or worse!).

Remember, nutrition is personal.

Lesson 2: Control Won't Save You (But It Will Burn You Out)
You started off learning about health and somewhere along the way, it turned into a mission to bio hack yourself into immortality. Nobody wins that game.

TRY THIS: Check in with yourself: Are you making decisions from fear or nourishment? Are you fuelling your body or trying to control the uncontrollable?

REMINDER: Trust will take you further than fear ever will.

CHAPTER ELEVEN

The Day My Body Quit

*"When the mind won't slow down,
the body turns up the volume."*
(Sammy Barnett)

My relentless drive to do more finally collided with the limits of my mind and body. It forced me to face the fallout of an overstimulated, undernourished existence.

My body handed in its resignation.

Red Flags? I Ignored Them All

I had a manual on staying safe – but took it to the extreme. Anxiety was trying to protect me in the only way it knew how, but I wasn't giving it any feedback. I took every warning as fact, never questioning whether the threat was real. I never said, '*I hear you, but I've got this.*'

Up until this moment, my life was spent overachieving and ignoring my limits. Eventually, that would catch up with me in the most dramatic way possible – through my body.

At first, it started with sleep. The less I slept, the more anxious I became. The more anxious I became, the less I slept. By 3am, my brain had me convinced I needed to start my day – or prepare for the inevitable *hallucination hour* – because why not add spiders to my problems?

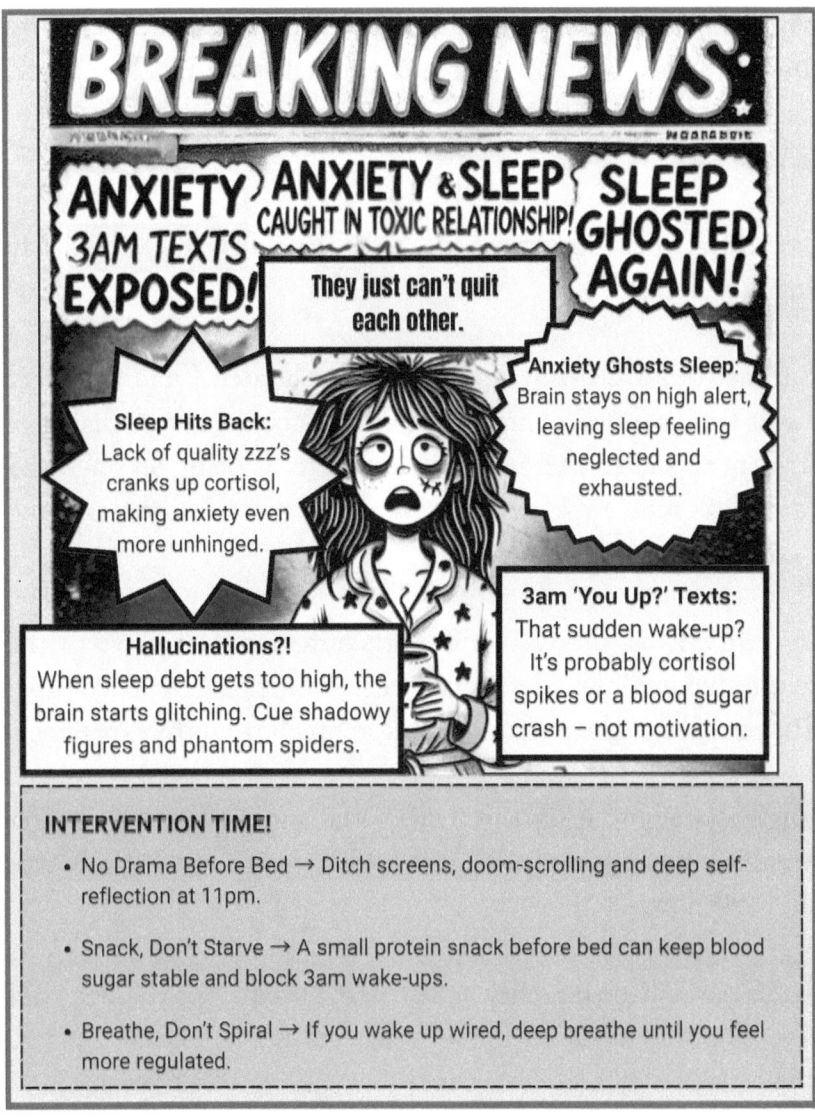

Anxiety and sleep were locked in a toxic relationship and my body was taking notes.

And one day, it had enough.

Enter: Adrenal exhaustion.

My new best friend – one that sucks the life out of you and drains any last drop of Tiger Juice. Exhaustion hit like a truck.

BAM!

I couldn't pick up my children. Stairs felt like Everest. My energy? Gone.

But instead of slowing down, I pushed harder. I had to. Three weeks from a fitness comp – the ultimate control test. A challenge that encapsulated everything: Diet, exercise, being on stage and sheer discipline. I told myself it was about growth, about proving I could master every variable.

In reality, I was also enjoying sports nutrition, fascinated by the science behind it all. The industry itself? Surprisingly welcoming. The people were lovely and I learnt so much from the experience.

But knowledge couldn't override exhaustion. I could no longer maintain my physique. No longer lift weights. My body was shutting down.

Turns out, when you refuse to listen, the teacher gets louder. And if that doesn't work? Well, then the teacher aggressively flips the whole desk over and makes sure you can't ignore it anymore.

Warning Signs Turned Warzone

First, I completely stopped menstruating (this didn't come back for almost a year). Then it was exhaustion. Then, weight loss. Then dizziness. The weird cramps I brushed off as 'training pains'.

But this? This was different.

A weird sensation on the right side of my body. A dull ache that wouldn't go away. I told my husband, *'Something doesn't feel right.'*

I was hyper-aware of my body sensations due to anxiety. I assumed it was a stomach ulcer. But I knew deep down that wasn't it. The stomach didn't sit on the right side of my body. My abs were out. I was ready to *rock* the stage.

But my body had other plans.

I drove myself to the hospital, convincing myself it was nothing serious. They took me straight in for tests. Then came the standard medical questions: *Drinking? Drugs? Living alone?*

At the time, it felt like an interrogation – like I was in an episode of *CSI*. Except the crime? My own body.

I told the doctor, *'I'm prepping for a fitness comp. I'm shredded. I'm about to go on stage.'*

And then he said it. The words I never saw coming.

'You have acute liver failure.'

The Diagnosis That Pulled The Brake

Everything inside me collapsed in an instant. My ears were ringing, my body felt weightless.

Acute Liver Failure.

The words bounced in my head. My body – the one I had pushed and fine-tuned – was done with me. And all I could think was…

'I almost didn't come. I almost ignored this. How long had I been killing myself while calling it <u>healthy</u>? How selfish of me!'

All the years chasing control, achievement, validation. But here I was, reduced to nothing but failing organs and a body that was done playing along.

'What does that mean?'

The answer was simple. It meant I was breaking down. And if I didn't stop, there would be nothing left of me to fix.

I thought liver failure was the ultimate wake-up call. It wasn't.

The real moment? That came later, when my five-year-old asked the question that would shatter me.

The only way to repair my liver – because, thankfully, it wasn't too far gone – was to start looking after myself the way it actually needed.

Although I was eating enough, I was tracking every macro, hitting 2,000 calories a day – my body was starving.

Turns out, my high-fat Keto diet plus chronic stress plus tanked cortisol was the perfect storm for liver burnout. Keto was meant to be *fuel-efficient* – but my body? It naturally struggles to break down fats. I have fat malabsorption, meaning my body wasn't properly digesting or absorbing the fats I was loading it up with. Without the right digestive enzymes to help, my liver was working overtime just to keep up.

NB: While Keto can be a useful tool for some, my specific case – made it a recipe for disaster. Fat malabsorption can be genetic, but it can also develop due to gut issues, low bile production, enzyme deficiencies, or chronic stress. For me? Probably all of the above.

And then there was stress.

Cortisol plays a key role in metabolism. It helps regulate blood sugar and energy production. Too much can overwhelm the liver. Too little? The system crashes.

The result? My liver had no backup, no support – just chronic overload.

And the biggest clue? I dreamt about carbs. My body wasn't just hungry – it was begging me for it. I had a fridge full of baked goods because cooking and smelling it was somewhat satisfying.

The Trophy I Almost Missed

Even after everything, I decided not to back out of the competition. I adjusted my plan – more nutritious liver loving foods.

And I stepped out on stage.

I had lost muscle definition. But I still placed third. The competition was over. Months of discipline, pushing, suffering – done.

Then, before I even had a second to process it, I felt a tiny hand grab mine. I looked down. My five-year-old, beaming with pride, his big blue eyes shining as he reached up for me.

'Congratulations Mummy!'

Then, with pure innocence, he asked the question that shattered me more than any diagnosis ever could.

'Can we have you back now?'

I felt the breath leave my body. My chest tightened.

I hadn't been gone for days or weeks. I had been gone for months. Physically there, mentally absent. And he had noticed. He had been waiting for me.

Tears blurred my vision. I crouched down, hands on his tiny shoulders. Guilt crashing over me. He wanted me to sit with him. Have meals with him. *Be present.*

The only trophy that mattered was right in front of me. Asking me to come home.

I had spent my life proving I was strong, capable, in control. But what if strength wasn't in pushing?

What if it was in finally letting go?

Healing – For Real, This Time

For the first time, I *asked for help*.

I reached out to an integrated doctor – someone who wouldn't just throw medication at me but actually *listen* to my story. I found her at a wellness event. The way she spoke and understood the body – it just clicked. She was the one who could help me.

When she ran tests, it was like checking under the hood of a car that had been running on fumes for years.

Thyroid? Sluggish.
Hormones? MIA.
Liver? Waving a white flag.
Adrenals? Staging a coup.

I was flatlined.

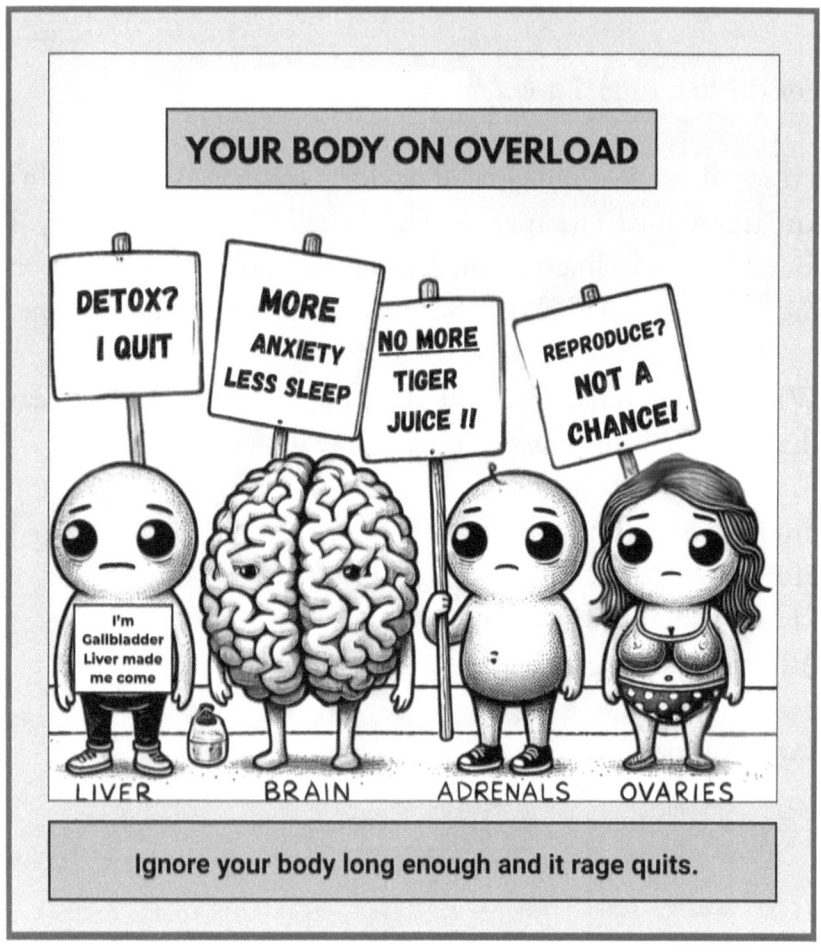

My body had been in survival for *so long* it wasn't even doing basic maintenance anymore. My skin was breaking out, hair falling out, body odour was noticeable and nails brittle and cracking. I was also experiencing menopausal symptoms like hot flushes. Fun times.

And to top it off, I found out I had the MTHFR gene variation – from both parents. And no, that doesn't stand for *'Mother F***er'* – although some days it really feels like it. I call it that anyway – in Samuel L Jackson's voice, of course.

What it actually means? My body struggles to convert folate (a B vitamin) into its usable form because of a glitch in my enzyme called methylenetetrahydrofolate reductase (yeah, try saying that fast three times). This enzyme is responsible for methylation, a process that affects detoxing, making neurotransmitters and overall nervous system function. Fabulous.

Not everyone with *MTHFR* experiences symptoms, but in my case – my body was struggling to keep up. It wasn't just a genetic variation sitting quietly in the background, it was actively impacting how I processed nutrients, regulated stress and detoxified.

Basically, my body isn't just struggling – it is biochemically wired to work harder at things like clearing toxins, regulating stress and producing feel-good chemicals.

Well, that explains a lot! I had spent my whole life following general health advice meant for *other* people – assuming what worked for them would work for me.

But now? I was finally figuring out *MY* body. Not a textbook case. Not a research paper. Just *me*.

I was given a gun at birth. And I'd spent my whole life loading it – stress, diet, lack of sleep. All I needed was the right *trigger*.

And I pulled it.

When 'Healthy' Made Me Worse

I thought I was doing everything right.

I was taking supplements, following all the expert advice, reading research papers like they were bedtime stories (seriously). But the very things I thought were *healing* me were actually making me *worse*.

Turns out, just because something is labelled 'healthy' doesn't mean it's good for *you*.

For me, taking the wrong form of B vitamins – without realising my body couldn't process them properly – felt like throwing fuel on an already anxious fire. For some people, they thrive on this form. My body? Not so much…Hello, crying in the shower for no reason.

Doctors had offered me anxiety meds before, which I know help many people in the short-term. But based on how my body reacted to medication in the past, I wanted to explore a different approach. For me, working in with my integrated doctor to find the right supplement forms made all the difference.

I wanted to do this *naturally*. But my previous natural approach had backfired.

I had completely missed one of the *biggest* factors in healing – it's not one-size-fits-all. And that included digestion. While others around me seemed to eat without a second thought, my body was running a different program – one wired for survival, not nourishment.

Digest or Run – Your Body Can't Do Both

Ever tried eating a salad while being chased by a tiger? No? Well, my body *thought* I had.

Digestion isn't a priority when your nervous system thinks you're in danger. Instead of breaking down food, your body diverts blood flow away from the digestive system and into your arms and legs – getting you ready to run for your life.

Those 'butterflies' in your stomach? That's your nervous system redirecting blood away from digestion toward the muscles in your extremities – preparing you to run. Great for escaping danger. Terrible for absorbing nutrients.

Short-term stress won't completely shut down digestion, but chronic stress? That's when your gut takes a serious hit:

- Stomach acid? Suppressed.
- Digestive enzymes? MIA.
- Nutrient absorption? LOL, no.

I could eat the *most* perfect diet in the world, but my body didn't care. It was too focused on survival to worry about breaking down a green goddess bowl of nutrients.

When survival mode kicks in, the body *prioritises* resources.

Beating heart? *Essential.*
Hair, nails, digestion? *Not so much.*

This is something I teach in my nutrition workshops – how to switch on the digestive system before eating. Whether it's through deep breathing, mindfulness, having a giggle or simply pausing before a meal, we can signal safety to the body and get digestion back online. It's one of the simplest, most powerful tools we have – and it's free. Try it before your next meal: pause, breathe and give your body a moment to catch up. Your gut will thank you.

Because you can't digest food while running from a tiger – even if the 'tiger' is just an email from John.

And to top it off, the foods I thought were saving me were actually making things worse. My digestive system is on the shorter side – which meant giant, fibre-packed salads weren't my friend. I needed small, nutrient-dense, partially cooked meals throughout the day. Not raw kale that my gut treated like a full-scale invasion.

It's not a one size fits all approach.

But instead of accepting that food alone wasn't the answer, I did what any overachiever would do – I went into full fix-it mode… again.

Information Overload

Even after everything, I still didn't *slow down*. I wasn't running just from death anymore, I was 'fixing' what I had broken. Putting myself back together so I could be a present mum again.

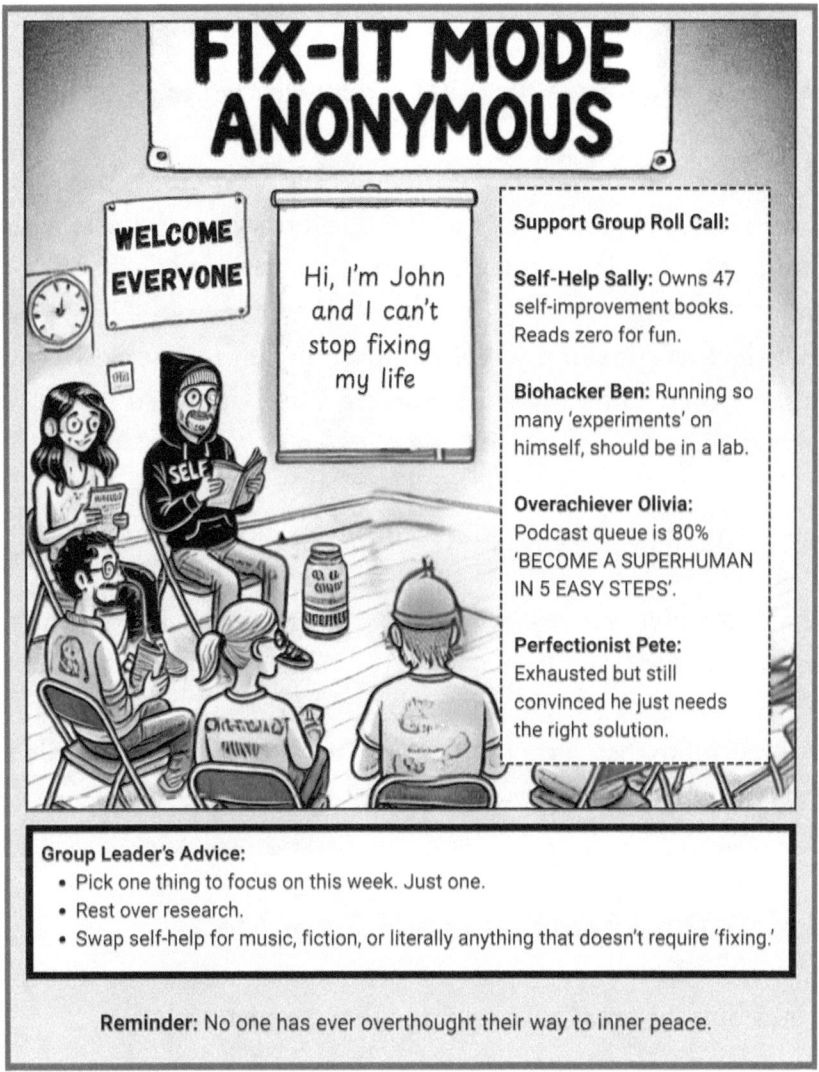

With the help of my new integrated doctor, I spiralled into researching the 'right' foods and supplements for my body. I had the ultimate blueprint now.

Each new podcast gave me a dopamine hit – then decision fatigue. I wasn't healthier – just buried under contradictions.

For the first time, I stopped trying to fix myself.

And you would not believe it. I actually felt better.

I swapped self-help books for fiction (*The Seven Sisters* series by Lucinda Riley saved me). I replaced information podcasts with music and dancing, something I had always loved.

For the first time in my life, I allowed myself to just exist. The more I tried to fix myself, the worse I felt. The need to know everything was making me *overstimulated*.

So, for the first time, I had a real conversation with anxiety:

'*I'll stop giving you new information. Let's just integrate what we already know.*'

And just like that, a tiny shift. A pause in the noise. But while I was learning to slow down, my work was speeding up.

I Had The Answers – Just Not For Me

I was busy in my clinic, helping other women heal.

At first, it seemed simple – heal the gut, lifestyle changes, tweak their diet, address sensitivities, correct deficiencies and watch them improve. And they did…for a while. But any stressor – a hard month, toxic conversations, bullying – could send them right back to square one.

That frustrated me.

I wanted them to have lasting healing. I wanted them to feel alive.

I was pouring everything into my clients, carrying the weight of their health concerns as if I could heal them myself. But what I learnt over time?

As a nutritionist, you don't heal people.

You give them the tools to heal themselves.

Clinic became lighter. And I also knew… *I* needed more tools.

I needed to understand how stress, trauma and the nervous system were affecting their health – and of course their food choices. I had to teach them how to fish, not just hand them the rod. This would be my next adventure.

The Hardest Lesson to Learn

For years, I thought anxiety was my teacher. And in many ways, it was. It led me to study the human body, to uncover the connections between food, stress and healing. Without it, I never would have gained the knowledge that now helps me guide other women on their own journeys.

It wasn't just something to manage – it was pointing me toward my purpose.

But anxiety wasn't the final authority on my life. It was just one voice in the room.

And honestly?

It was time for it to take some notes.

Because here's the truth – healing isn't about doing more. It's about doing less. You cannot integrate when you are constantly consuming. You cannot heal while stuck in the cycle of fixing.

The people who have truly done the most healing? They're not reading self-help books anymore.

They're living. They're in the moment. They're listening to their bodies.

That is healing.

That is what saved me. And I hope, in some way, it saves you too. Because, at the end of it all, I was about to learn something I had never done before.

Be still.

Healing wasn't another goal to tick off. It was the opposite of everything I had ever known. Instead of pushing harder, I had to surrender. Instead of researching more, I had to feel more. Instead of controlling everything, I had to trust my body to heal – if I let it.

Class is over, anxiety. I am the teacher now.

ANXIETY CHEAT SHEET: What You Need to Know

If you don't listen to the whispers, your body will start screaming.

Lesson 1: Your Body Doesn't Care About Your Deadlines
You can ignore exhaustion, hunger, stress – but your body won't.

TRY THIS: When your body whispers – fatigue, headaches, bloating – listen before it starts screaming. Your body isn't betraying you. It's doing its best – sometimes it just needs a little help.

Lesson 2: The Trophies That Matter Aren't the Ones You Chase
I was chasing the wrong trophies.

TRY THIS: Look at where you're putting your energy – would your future self say it was worth it? Ask yourself: *Am I running toward something meaningful, or am I just running?* The most important trophies are often the ones already in front of you.

REMINDER: Your body isn't the enemy – it's the messenger.

CHAPTER TWELVE

The Woo-Woo Awakening

"It's not the perfect parts that shape you, it's the cracked ones that let the light pour in."
(Sammy Barnett)

I thought I was just exploring new ways to heal – until the universe cracked me wide open and showed me things I never could have imagined.

When I ditched research papers, I started exploring things I'd always side-eyed. I was science-based, but deep down, I knew there was still so much we didn't understand.

Curious but sceptical – I walked into the woo.

I had friends deeply connected to spiritual practices. I wasn't about to strip naked under a full moon, but…something was there. So, I dipped my toes in:

- Chinese medicine
- Reiki
- NLP (Neuro-Linguistic Programming)
- Hypnotherapy
- Breathwork

Out of everything I'd learnt, the breath had always been my number one tool for regulating my nervous system. It's free, always available and yet so many of us forget to use it.

Because if a tiger *really* were chasing you, stopping to take a deep breath would get you eaten. But when you do pause – when you take that slow, mindful inhale – you're telling your body, *There is no tiger. You are safe.* And sometimes, that's the most powerful message you can send.

Breathwork:
Nature's Free Nervous System Upgrade
(No drugs. No guru robes. Just you, your lungs and a little science.)

So, you think you already know how to breathe? But did you know changing how you breathe can literally rewire your nervous system?

What's Actually Happening?

- Vagus nerve activates sending 'We're safe now' signals to your body.
- Oxygen and CO2 balance sharpening focus and chilling anxiety.
- Stored stress and trauma releases from deep within the nervous system.
- A natural high is triggered – no shady back-alley deals required.

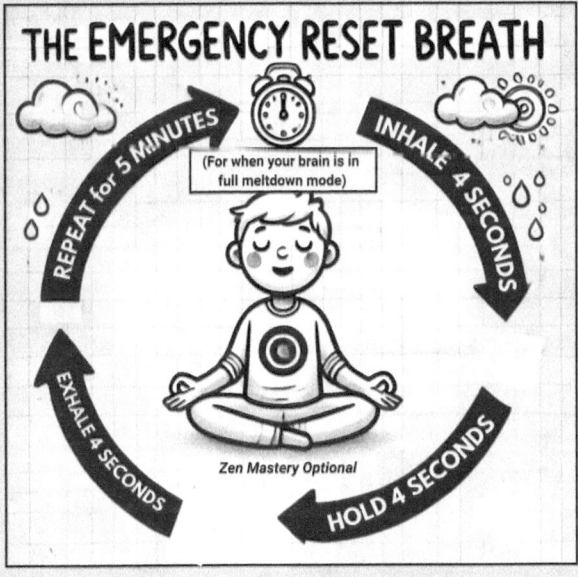

What I didn't realise about breathwork is that it can be so powerful that you become *The Last Airbender* – real life.

I was not prepared for what was about to unfold.

In the days leading up to the breathwork session at a course I had signed up to, things started shifting. Memories surfaced. Emotions bubbled up. And when the session finally began, it hit me like a tidal wave.

I thought I was just clearing out some nervous system cobwebs. Regulating my stress, calming my body. You know, basic human maintenance. But breathwork doesn't just clear out today's stress – it cracks open the vault.

And in that vault?

A backlog of pain that didn't even start with me.

Generations of it.

My mother's. My grandmother's. The weight of survival, of unspoken grief passed down like a family heirloom. The things they never processed – I was carrying.

And now, through breath, it was surfacing.

I walked into that session thinking I was just stressed out, trying to hack my nervous system. I left realising I was the emotional processing plant for my entire bloodline.

Then, in the middle of this wild breathing journey, it happened.

In that moment, it felt like I connected with something beyond myself – my lineage, my history, maybe even the women who came before me.

My ancestors.

Yep! My ancestors! Things are about to get weird.

They had a message for me – one that would shake me to the core.

'Anxiety isn't a curse. It's a gift.'

And then they said…

'YOU ARE A WITCH!'

The Witchy Revelation

I was *not* expecting this. And honestly? I wasn't sure whether to believe it.

I was deep in another plane of existence, feeling everything so intensely. And then…I saw them. A coven of witches. They were my ancestors. Some held my hands. Others circling around me, chanting, dancing.

I physically *felt* them grasp my hands – even though, in this world, nothing was there.

And they told me…

'Anxiety isn't a curse. It's a gift. A tool. A power to connect with myself and the world around me. A tool to heal those that walk beside me.'

They said I was meant to teach and heal.

Anxiety was never meant to destroy me. It was meant to guide me.

'You are part of a powerful coven of witches.'

And I lay there, thinking…

WHAT. THE. ACTUAL. F-

I had never considered anything like this before. I was logical, science-based, grounded.

Sure, my mum named me after Samantha from *Bewitched,* but this? This was something else. The witches weren't just dancing – they were midwifing generational trauma. Yep. I was literally screaming, pushing – minus the actual baby and blood.

But I could sense something leaving my body and I remember screaming, *'GET OUT, GET OUT!'*

It was like I had no control of my body. This was just happening – and I was there for the experience.

But after the pain…I felt lighter, freer. I could feel my body lifting, projecting upward, as if I were expanding beyond myself. A white light filled the room, radiating outward, surrounding everything. It wasn't just inside me – I could feel it pushing out, a powerful force spilling into the space around me. It was as if, in that moment, I wasn't just releasing my own pain – I was sending healing energy into the room, into everyone around me.

When I came to, we had a moment to share our experience within the group. A man who was lying near me said, '*I had the strangest experience. There were a bunch of ladies dancing around me. I have no idea why.*'

I froze.

I hadn't told anyone about my experience yet. And yet, he saw them too.

We talked afterward. When I asked his ancestry, he said his family were from a specific part of the world.

Goosebumps.

Because that was exactly where *my* ancestors were from, too.

The High That Led to the Crash

For the next few days, I felt *incredible*.

I was light. Free. Energised. I could see and feel things on a whole new level.

I was 'Neo', fresh off the red pill, watching the world in HD. Yes, another Keanu reference.

I had cracked the code – just by breathing. I had upgraded my nervous system to a whole new level. No drugs. No external chemicals. Just me and my own lungs flipping my consciousness inside out.

Breathwork flooded my body with oxygen, boosting my brain chemistry. It was like hitting a hidden 'unlock' button – my body buzzing, my awareness cranked up to eleven. Some people say breathwork can trigger deep emotional releases, heightened awareness, even full-blown visions. All I know is…something cracked open.

Spiritual awakenings are chemical, too – dopamine and serotonin spike, then crash.

I had opened up something I wasn't ready for.

Generational weight came rushing in.

It's called 'spiritual bypassing' – opening too fast without the tools to process it. In the book, *The Body Keeps the Score (2014)*, Dr Bessel van der Kolk explains how trauma isn't just in the mind – it lives in the body. If we unlock it without integration, it can knock us sideways.

And it did.

I had taken the red pill, but instead of taking me further into the *Matrix*, it propelled me back into reality.

Only this place was dark.

Strange.

And terrifying.

The underworld. The emotions. The overwhelm. The *intensity* of it all.

I felt watched. Like my ancestors were following me around, whispering to me.

I thought I had done my work. I had used tools like 'Timeline Therapy'. But this? This was another layer. It felt like I was 11 years old again. Full of fear, it followed me everywhere.

I went from being the most connected I'd ever been…to feeling like I didn't even want to be on this planet anymore.

Disconnected, paranoid – like everyone was against me. A burden with nothing to offer.

My life was *fine*. I had *nothing* to complain about.

That didn't change the fact that I felt like I was drowning.

The Darkest Night

Guilt crept in with every wave of sadness.

I knew others had been through much worse. Were still going through worse.

I remembered Holocaust survivor Edith Eger's book, *The Choice: Embrace the Possible (2017)*. She wrote about how pain is deeply personal – how comparing suffering doesn't lessen your own, it only undermines your healing.

But damn, it's hard not to compare.

'Other people have it worse. Your life is fine. Stop being dramatic.'

I kept telling myself that. Dismissing my pain as if acknowledging it made me ungrateful.

But pain doesn't work like that. It's not a competition. There's no Suffering Olympics where only the person with the worst trauma earns the right to feel hurt.

And yet, no matter how much I tried to rationalise it, I still felt like I was drowning.

I didn't know what to do with all of it – the heaviness, the sadness, the feeling like I had opened something inside me I couldn't close.

One night in the kitchen, I sobbed while my husband held me. He knew I wasn't okay, but he didn't know what else to do. He is a fixer.

I wasn't having a breakthrough or a lesson – I was just lost in it. I had no idea how to fix it myself. I just knew I couldn't keep doing it alone. For me, that meant finding people who could hold space. For others, it might mean therapy, community, or something entirely different.

Healing isn't one-size-fits-all.

And what made it worse?

I didn't even know feeling this way after a spiritual awakening was normal.

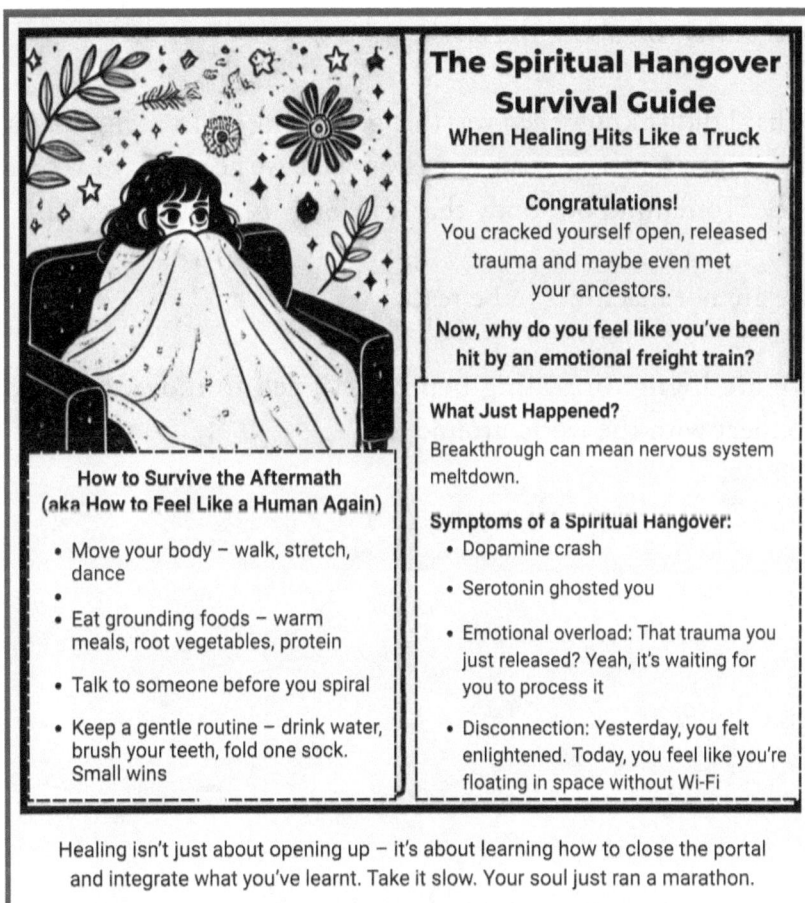

Breathwork shakes your system. Grounding helps, but some may need professional support to fully integrate the experience.

I expected relief, maybe even clarity. Instead, I felt more anxious than before. Anxiety wasn't the villain here. It was the aftershock.

I needed to sit with it. Because sometimes, the best lessons don't come from the breakthrough itself…but from what happens after.

You hear about *healing, transcendence, spiritual awakenings*. No one warns you about the crash.

What I didn't know then was that grounding is just as important as healing. When we crack ourselves open, we need a way to come back. To remind our body that it belongs *here*, on this earth.

We are not machines to be reset.

We are living, breathing beings designed to move, feel and connect with the world around us.

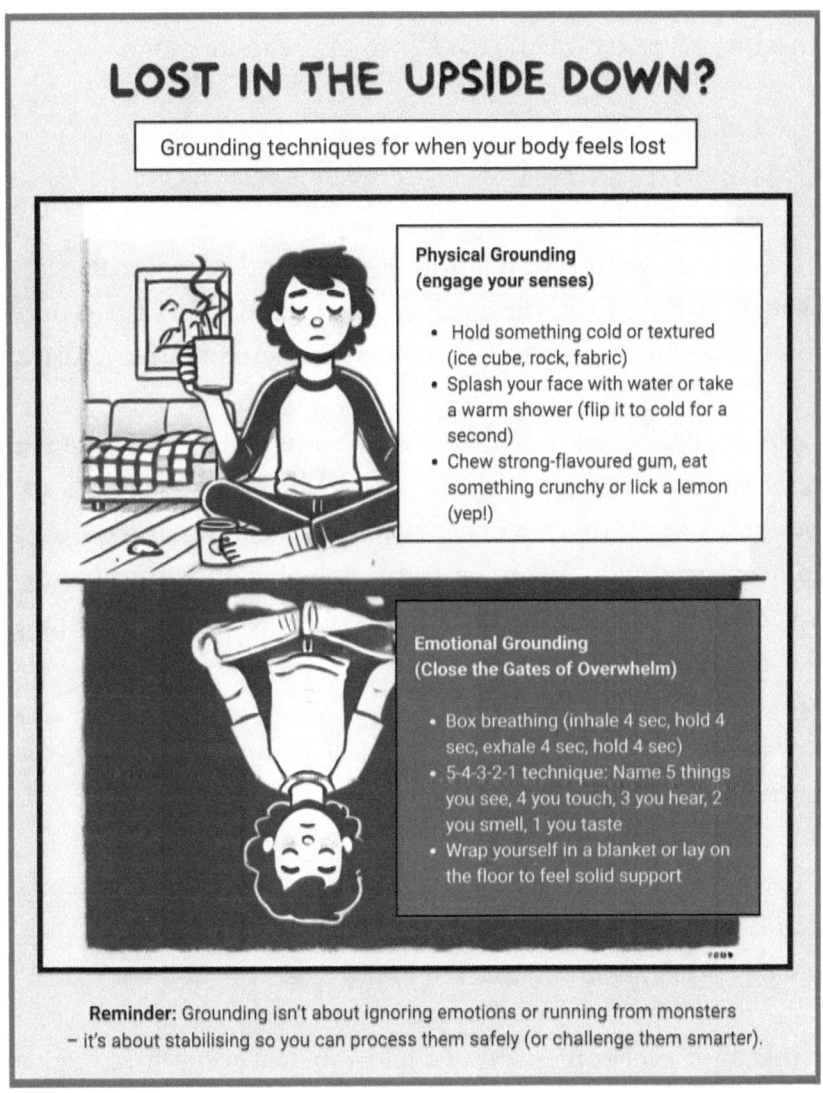

When you dive deep into yourself, you need a way to return. To feel your feet on the ground, your breath in your lungs, your place in this world. Healing isn't about blowing your life wide open – it's about putting yourself back together in a way that makes sense.

But I couldn't see that yet. All I knew was that I was spiralling and I was furious I had been left to figure it out alone.

Closing The Portal

I didn't feel safe in my own skin. Every sound felt sharper, every shadow darker. Even the smell of sage – something I had once found comforting – now sent my nervous system into overdrive.

Looking back now, one of the only things that made me feel safe was the sound of my sister's voice. Maybe it was familiarity, maybe it was the rhythm of her words, maybe it was just knowing someone was there. When everything else felt unpredictable, her voice was a tether – something constant in the chaos. So, I rang her every hour, on the hour.

I was stuck between two worlds. Too open, too raw, too untethered.

That's when I was referred to a healer. Someone who, apparently, could help me close the darn portal I had accidentally kicked open.

I told him everything. How I had touched something bigger than me and now I didn't know how to exist in the world I had known before. How I felt like I had unlocked a door I wasn't meant to open – only to realise I had no idea how to shut it.

He listened without flinching, like he'd heard stories like mine a thousand times before. And then, he got to work.

He didn't just *close* a portal. He brought me back to myself.

He told me something that changed my idea of healing:

'Healing isn't just deep work – it's also found in joy, connection and safety.'

At the time, I was recently taught that healing meant tearing yourself apart, digging through every trauma, facing every dark corner of your soul.

But what if it didn't?

What if healing could be gentle as well?

What if it could happen in moments of safety, joy and connection – instead of just in the depths of suffering?

He guided me through grounding rituals, pulling my energy back into my own body. It didn't happen instantly. But by the end of our session, I felt…*somewhat* solid again.

I could breathe without feeling like I was being watched. I could stand without feeling like I was falling into the abyss. It would be a long time before I dipped my toes back into the spiritual side of healing.

I wasn't ready. I needed time. I needed to trust my body again.

And I needed more support.

The Man Who Helped Me Cry

I reached out to a friend, an emotions coach for women. When I told him what was happening, he offered me a free session out of pure kindness.

In that session, something shifted.

For once, anxiety wasn't screaming to be heard. I could sit with it, without letting it take over. In this moment it didn't feel like an enemy, but as a guide. A light.

The witches were right.

And just as I was beginning to make peace with that, my emotions coach hit me with a truth bomb:

'You intellectualise everything', he said. *'And you use humour to cover your emotions.'*

Damn. Called out!

He was right.

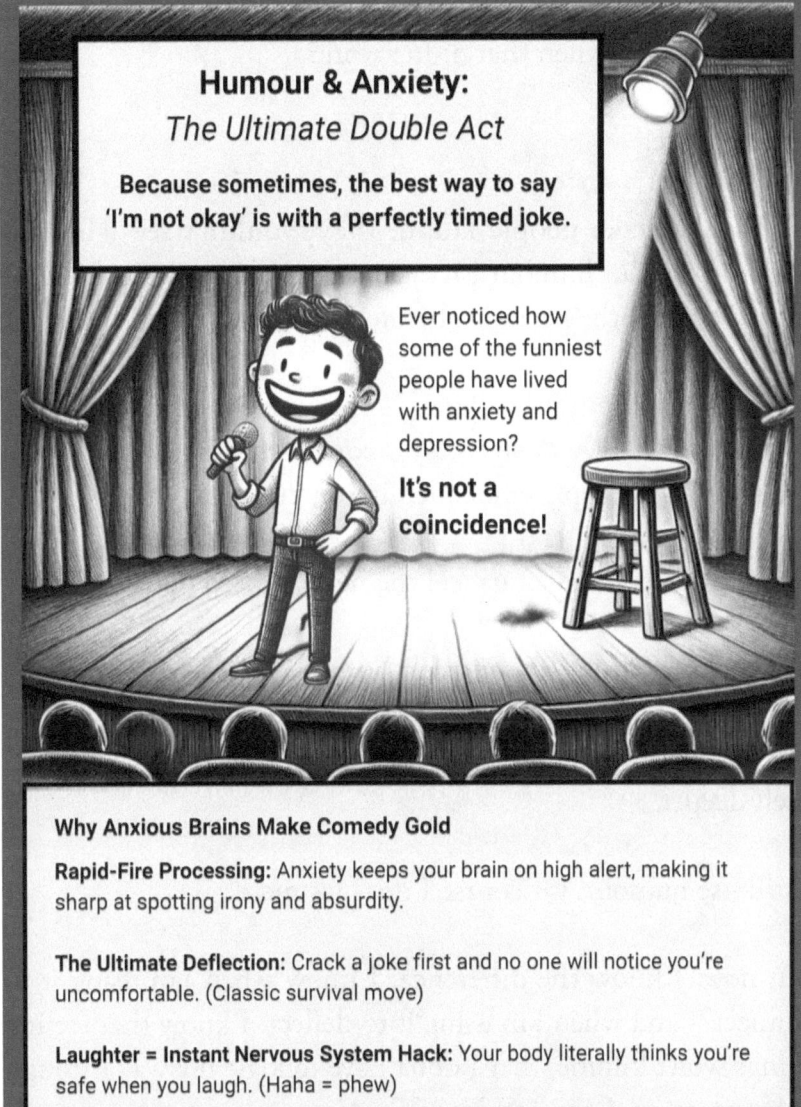

Humour & Anxiety:
The Ultimate Double Act

Because sometimes, the best way to say 'I'm not okay' is with a perfectly timed joke.

Ever noticed how some of the funniest people have lived with anxiety and depression?

It's not a coincidence!

Why Anxious Brains Make Comedy Gold

Rapid-Fire Processing: Anxiety keeps your brain on high alert, making it sharp at spotting irony and absurdity.

The Ultimate Deflection: Crack a joke first and no one will notice you're uncomfortable. (Classic survival move)

Laughter = Instant Nervous System Hack: Your body literally thinks you're safe when you laugh. (Haha = phew)

Here's the Catch: Buried feelings ferment.

Next time you crack a joke about something painful, pause. Am I laughing because it's funny, or because I'm avoiding something real? Humour helps – but healing happens when we feel, too.

I had spent my life thinking my way out of feeling. Logic was my shield. And when that didn't work?

Crack a joke.

If I could make people laugh, they wouldn't see what lay underneath. But humour isn't just a punchline – it's a shield. A way to control the narrative before it controls you.

As Susan Cain put it in *Quiet*, *"The pressure to entertain, to sell ourselves, and never to be visibly anxious keeps ratcheting up"* – a pressure that's deeply embedded in our culture.

No wonder so many of us feel the need to keep up the act.

But here's the thing about using humour to hide pain:

The weight of what's underneath doesn't go away – it just buries itself deeper.

I still use humour. Of course I do – it's me.

But now, I know the difference. I know when I'm using it to connect – and when I'm using it to deflect. I know that feeling things won't kill me, that I don't have to logic my way through every emotion. I can just let it be.

The comedians we've lost to mental health struggles weren't weak. They carried so much weight while making others laugh. But knowing it and feeling it? Two very different things.

That's where the emotions coach came in.

In that session, he held space for me.

And I cried.

And cried.

And cried.

For weeks, I cried.

I cried for the little girl inside me who had been ignored for so long. I had spent life trying to protect her, not listening to her.

I cried for the version of me that was always trying to *prove* something.

I cried for the exhaustion, the stress, the perfectionism.

I cried for the people I had pulled away from, not because I didn't love them, but because I didn't know how to hold them *and* hold myself at the same time.

I cried for the friendships I let fade, the moments I missed, the times I had to choose healing over showing up.

I cried for the guilt of putting myself first – even when I knew I had to.

I cried for everything.

And that was when the real healing started.

ANXIETY CHEAT SHEET: What You Need To Know

Or:

Things I Wish I'd Known Before Accidentally Summoning My Ancestors

Lesson 1: Healing Doesn't Have to Feel Like an Exorcism
Play. Rest. Laugh. Experience joy without feeling like you have to earn it. Healing doesn't have to be *Stranger Things*-level weird.

TRY THIS: If you've been in the trenches of deep healing work, balance it out with something light. Play music, go outside, watch something that makes you laugh. Not every breakthrough requires a breakdown.

Sometimes, healing happens when you let yourself be happy.

Lesson 2: A Breakdown Might Just be A Breakthrough
Is it proof that something may be shifting?

TRY THIS: *What if this feeling isn't a setback, but a sign of change?* Instead of fighting it, give yourself space to adjust. Treat it like a nervous system reboot – your body is catching up to the work you've done.

Healing can be a dance between the light and dark.

REMINDER: Healing isn't about escaping yourself – it's about coming home to who you've always been.

CHAPTER THIRTEEN

Learning to Sit Before We Fly

*"Rebuilding doesn't always start with action.
Sometimes, it begins with the courage to
sit in discomfort and finally face what
you've been running from."*
(Sammy Barnett)

I had always been the one charging ahead, but now I was stuck – trapped in a cocoon of uncertainty, watching life move while I stayed still.

I'd been sitting in the ickiness for a while. My husband, friends and family were worried. I was consumed by guilt and shame, standing at the edge of a crossroad, unsure which way to go.

Should I return to what I know or step into the unknown?

Anxiety spun me in circles, an over-caffeinated teacher yelling, *'Hurry up!'* while I was still trying to read the darn book. I pushed back. *'Not yet. We need to wait.'*

And so, I sat. I let the discomfort wash over me instead of rushing to the next thing. Anxiety hated it – nagging, poking, pacing the room. But when the time was right, that same anxious energy that once held me captive became the force that set me free. And for that, I had to thank it.

I used every tool I had used in clinic – only this time, on myself. In a way that felt safe.

Flipping the Board

Going back to my old life didn't sit right. It made me more uneasy.

So, I did it – I flipped the *Monopoly* board over and said, *'I'm out!'* I was making space for what was next. (And yes, I *am* a board flipper. Just ask my husband.)

Letting go wasn't just about walking away from work. It was releasing guilt, shame and the belief that I had to fight myself.

People said I was brave for throwing away everything I'd built. And honestly, I was. But it was also necessary.

I didn't just walk away from clinic – I realigned with what truly lit me up. My work evolved into something even more impactful, where I could bring my knowledge to wider audiences in a way that felt energising, not draining.

Rearranging the Puzzle

Despite my success, my work at the time didn't align with my core values.

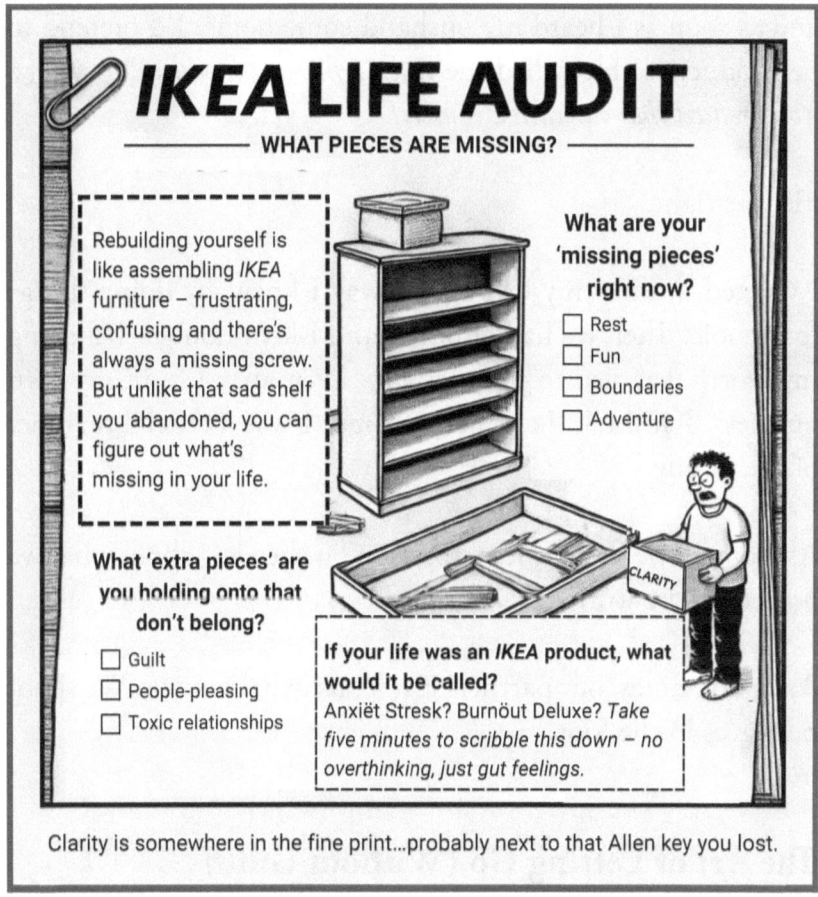

For me? *Fun. Family. Freedom.* I was too busy fixing everyone, including myself.

So, I shut down my podcast. Cleared my external commitments.

And weirdly enough, COVID-19 hit just before all this happened. It was like the universe handed me a permission slip: *Take a break. Also, here's a global pandemic so you don't feel guilty about it.*

I wasn't just a doer – I was a compulsive doer. I'd sit on the couch and as soon as I heard my husband come home, I'd pretend to be productive. He called me out: *'I never ask you to do things. You created that narrative yourself.'*

He was right.

I wanted to show my love in the way I knew, by doing things for people. Then we had children and I kept doing – believing my worth was tied to productivity. Even after I built my own business, I still felt like I had to *prove* I was a crucial member of the family.

As women, we create these stories in our heads – about what we *must* do to be worthy.

And sometimes, our partners just let us live them out. We shoot ourselves in the foot.

The Art of Letting Go (Without Guilt)

I started delegating.

I hired a cleaner. This unearthed something even deeper – a wound I didn't expect. Spending money on something I could do myself felt *wrong*. I had a terrible relationship with money, one built on guilt, scarcity and the belief that every dollar spent needed to be justified. Letting go of that was tough. But that story? That's for another book.

I stopped cooking every meal. Let my children fend for themselves in the kitchen. Okay, not full *Lord of the Flies*, but they did learn the horror of running out of bowls before realising the dishwasher exists.

I know not everyone can outsource everything, but for me, delegating what I *could*, freed up energy for things that actually mattered – things no one else could do for me.

I also had to accept that food was only *one* piece of the health puzzle. I used to obsess over every ingredient. Turns out, nourishment is also in laughter – even over pizza.

I get to make a choice. I know how foods make me feel and I can choose accordingly. The body is incredibly good at healing. It just needs the *right* environment – not just the right food.

When Doing is Hiding

I started noticing that my need to stay busy wasn't about productivity – it was about *avoiding emotions.*

Anxiety: The Best TEACHER You Never Asked For

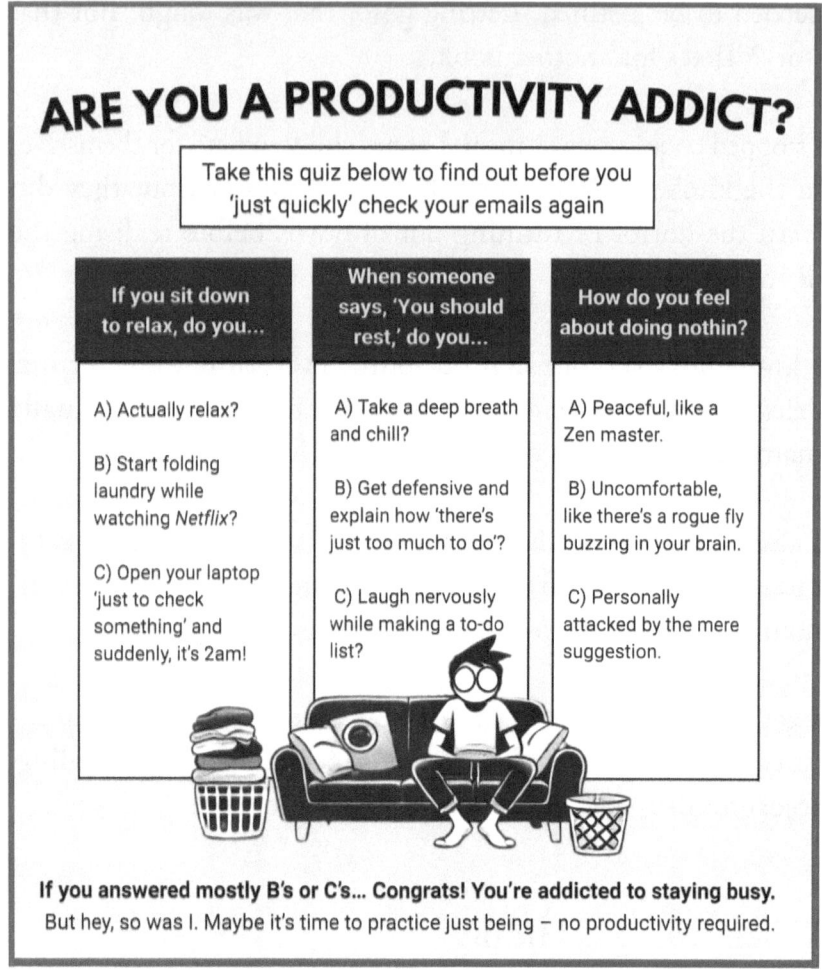

We stay busy to avoid feeling. But stillness is where healing happens.

Feeling it All: The Hardest Step in Healing

For the first time, I let myself *feel*.

Fear. Sadness. Abandonment. Loneliness. Confusion. The weight of my own expectations.

Instead of overanalysing, instead of spinning false narratives, I just sat with it.

Anxiety had been protecting me all these years. That panic? That gut-wrenching feeling? It was my body saying, *'I've got you.'*

I started talking. Sharing stories I had buried – guilt, regrets, old wounds. Apologising where I needed to.

And little by little, I healed.

We don't heal to go back to who we once were. We heal to become something stronger.

When we allow ourselves to sit in raw emotions, we acknowledge our humanity. *We are meant to feel.* Yet so many of us have become robotic, viewing crying and sensitivity as weaknesses.

They're not.

Allowing yourself to release emotions – without performing for others – is healing. When we cry, we're letting go of things our body has been holding onto.

I realised I didn't need fixing. When I sat in the ickiness, I reconnected with myself. Anxiety wasn't the enemy – it was trying to protect me.

I just needed to stop fighting it.

And yet, even as I made peace with my emotions, my body still felt 'off' – like it was running on a different time zone than my life.

Your Brain is Jetlagged and You Haven't Even Travelled

We think we're in control – that we can push through exhaustion with coffee and willpower. But no matter how much we try to outsmart biology, we are still wired like cavemen.

Our body's internal clock – the Suprachiasmatic Nucleus (SCN) – is the 'John Wick' of timekeeping. Mess with it and it will *definitely* come for you... Probably with insomnia and an existential crisis. Science shows that when we disrupt natural rhythms, everything from digestion to mental clarity takes a hit.

This tiny brain region controls sleep, hormones, digestion and mood. It's designed to sync with *natural* light, guiding us through cycles of energy and rest.

But modern life? It hijacks the system. Artificial light, erratic mealtimes and stress leave us wired at night, exhausted in the morning and disconnected from hunger cues.

Healing isn't just about sleep or food – it's about how we absorb life itself. When we fight against our body's natural cycles, everything becomes harder: digestion, energy, mental clarity, even our ability to feel calm.

Real healing doesn't come from forcing or fixing – it comes from realigning – listening instead of overriding. Trusting that your body knows what it's doing when given the right conditions.

So what are those 'right' conditions? Our internal clock – that circadian rhythm – runs the show. It doesn't just control sleep; it regulates the release of hormones like cortisol (wake up juice) and melatonin (sleep juice). It tells you when to feel hungry, when to poop, when to rest and when to focus. And when we sync with it, life flows better.

One of the simplest ways to realign? Let sunlight hit your eyes within 30 minutes of waking. In the evening, dim the lights to mimic sunset. Ever gone camping without screens or city lights? Your body slips back into rhythm like it never left. Even if life doesn't allow for a perfect natural schedule, you can mimic it – with sunrise clocks, blackout curtains and gentle routines. There's always a way to come at least 1% back to alignment.

Anxiety doesn't just come from overthinking – it comes from being out of sync with ourselves. When I stopped forcing my body to operate on stress and willpower and started working *with* it, everything shifted.

Less panic.

Less exhaustion.

Less feeling like I was at war with myself.

Maybe anxiety wasn't the problem. Maybe my disconnection was.

As a nutritionist, I once believed 'You are what you eat.' But the truth?

You are what you *absorb*.

And that goes beyond food.

Mindset Work Alone Isn't Enough

People often ask *'Where do I start? What do I eat? What do I need to do?'*

But healing isn't a checklist. And we love a good checklist – especially when we're anxious.

Anxiety doesn't need a to-do-list. It needs you to listen.

Cold plunges, therapy and journaling can be powerful – if they help you process, not just power through. The real breakthrough isn't in the ice bath. It's in what you do *afterwards*.

We don't heal by ticking off boxes. We heal by learning to listen to ourselves.

You can journal about self-love all day long, but if your nervous system is still in survival mode, those words won't land.

Yes, movement helps.

Yes, nutrition helps.

But if something deeper is going on – if there's an old wound whispering beneath all the noise – maybe it's time to stop *doing* and start *feeling*.

One of my biggest breakthroughs came when I stopped searching for answers and started *listening*. I truly believe life's struggles shape us. Every challenge has taught me something valuable – and the more I leaned into self-awareness and nervous system regulation, the more patterns I saw emerge.

I worked with and alongside incredible therapists. Therapy is an incredible tool. A therapist can hold space and offer insights, but true healing happens when we take that work into our daily lives. That had to come from me.

So I journaled.

Sometimes nonsense.

Other times, pure clarity.

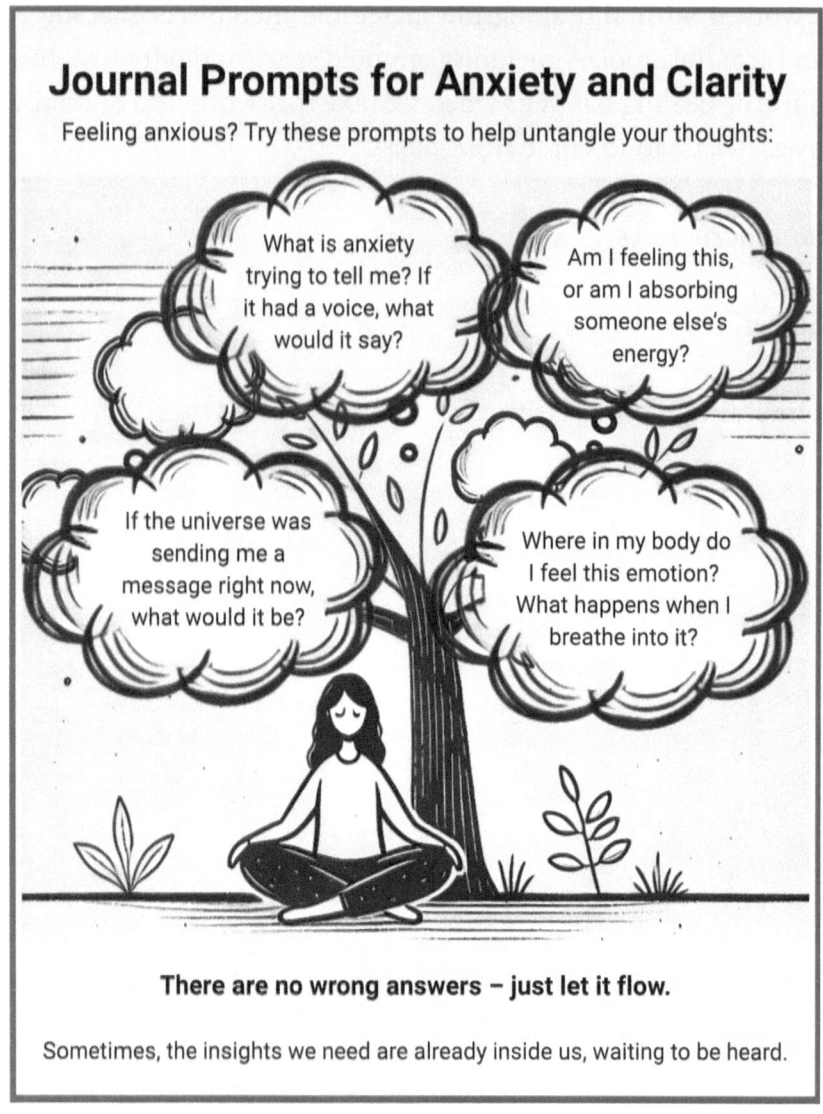

Connection is the Missing Link

When I felt comfortable in my skin again, I reconnected with something I'd loved since childhood – entertaining. Making people laugh. Lifting their spirits. That was healing.

The more I laughed and spread joy, the more I was letting anxiety know there weren't any tigers.

I wasn't just cracking jokes. I was making people feel seen and heard. And in doing so, I learnt something incredible.

We don't just exist alongside each other – we absorb each other's emotions, body language and nervous system signals. This is co-regulation. Our nervous systems sync up like Bluetooth.

Whether we realise it or not, we are constantly influencing and being influenced by the energy of those around us. Calm people ground us. Anxious people fry us. It's biology.

For years, anxiety convinced me healing was a solo mission. But a better lesson?

We heal in laughter.

We heal in connection.

We heal when we stop trying to be 'fixed' and start allowing ourselves to *be*.

From Clinic to Comedy

I used to dream of being a theme park character – until I pictured 'Daffy Duck' having a panic attack getting escorted out. Not a good look.

For years, I had been avoiding – avoiding death, avoiding fear, avoiding everything that *could* go wrong.

But instead of focusing on what could go wrong, I started focusing on *living*. You can't live if you're afraid to die.

I let go of the need to be perfect. Stopped caring so much about what people thought. And when I did, I started attracting my tribe. The people who got me. The ones who embraced me, quirks and all.

Before COVID-19, I had been running children's workshops, teaching nutrition in a fun, engaging and easy to grasp way. Breaking complex topics down for children came naturally to me. I had already been teaching my own children like this for years.

Then, COVID-19 hit. Everything paused. And in that stillness, I re-evaluated everything.

My clinic no longer felt like me.

So, I rebranded. Fun, light and aligned.

I let go of the rigid version of success I had clung to and allowed myself to build something that felt *right* for who I was in that moment.

I brought humour into my work. I wore silly hats. Ran fun digestion experiments. Parents started asking me to bring my workshops into corporate workplaces. And before I knew it, I was standing in front of suits – teaching them about gut health with *Mr Poo Hat* proudly perched on my head.

This was never the career path I mapped out, but because I gave myself the space to sit in the unknown, it unfolded naturally – better than I could have planned. Those solitary moments were not just a retreat, but also a wellspring of creativity and self-discovery. It is in these quiet times I find the space to dream and imagine.

Over time, I built something so unique and ridiculously fun, that the universe basically handed me a giant *'Keep going'* sign. I was nominated for *Jamie Oliver's Food Hero Award* and took out runner up in Australia. *The Wiggles* judging my work. Verdict? Brilliant.

I had built something unique, fun and fully aligned with who I was.

No more grinding. Just momentum, joy and purpose.

Becoming the Butterfly

No longer searching for validation. No longer afraid to be my full, quirky self.

People were drawn to my energy – not because I was trying to heal them, but because I was simply being me.

I had stepped fully into my power and it was *freeing*.

Rebuilding isn't about rushing toward the next version of yourself. It's about trusting that who you are becoming is already unfolding – one pause, one breath, one moment at a time.

And now, here's my challenge for you:

Stop.

Just for a moment.

Take a deep breath and sit in whatever *is* right now. No fixing, no forcing – just feeling.

Because sometimes, the most powerful thing you can do is...

Create space.

Space to listen.

Space to realign.

Space to let the next step reveal itself – rather than forcing one that isn't meant for you.

ANXIETY CHEAT SHEET:
What You Need To Know

Rebuilding starts with self-compassion. With sitting in discomfort. With letting go of perfectionism and most importantly, with learning to *live* the way YOU want to live!

Lesson 1: Anxiety Can Be Pushy
Is it yelling at you to move when you're *not ready yet?*

TRY THIS: Instead of letting anxiety rush you, ask: *Is this the right time to act, or do I need to wait and absorb?* When anxiety screams, *'DO SOMETHING!'* respond with, *'We're stretching first, calm down.'*

Sometimes, waiting *is* the breakthrough.

Lesson 2: Your Nervous System is Like a Wi-Fi Signal – Protect Your Connection
Your nervous system syncs up with the people around you, just like your phone automatically connects to Wi-Fi. Be mindful of your 'network.'

TRY THIS: When you feel anxious, do a Connection Audit. Who in your life makes you feel safe, understood and grounded? Spend more time with them.

Reminder: Surround yourself with people who help you feel stable.

CHAPTER FOURTEEN

Gifts of the Sensitive Soul

*"Anxiety isn't here to ruin you,
it's here to reroute you."* (Sammy Barnett)

To feel everything is overwhelming, but it also allows us to connect, create and heal.

Someone once told me that sensitivity is a weakness – that calling a child sensitive would somehow break them. But sensitivity isn't a weakness. It's a gift.

Sure, it means I might cry during commercials. I mean, *The Lion King* already emotionally wrecked me (I'm sure you remember the death of 'Mufasa'). But this also means I see beauty where others miss it. Fair trade, I say.

Have you ever *felt* a sunset? I have.

More Than A Feeling

Sensitivity allows me to experience the world so deeply – the good, the bad and the breathtakingly beautiful. It's what helps me pick up on small shifts in energy, the unspoken emotions lingering in a crowded room.

I've always been the person who instinctively walks over to someone who looks uneasy, offering comfort and, let's be real, probably an awkward joke to lighten the mood, too. Sensitivity helps me connect.

But it's also a challenge. When you absorb *everything* – people's emotions, energy, even the subtle tension in the air – it can drain you. Without boundaries, it can consume you. And for a long time, I let it.

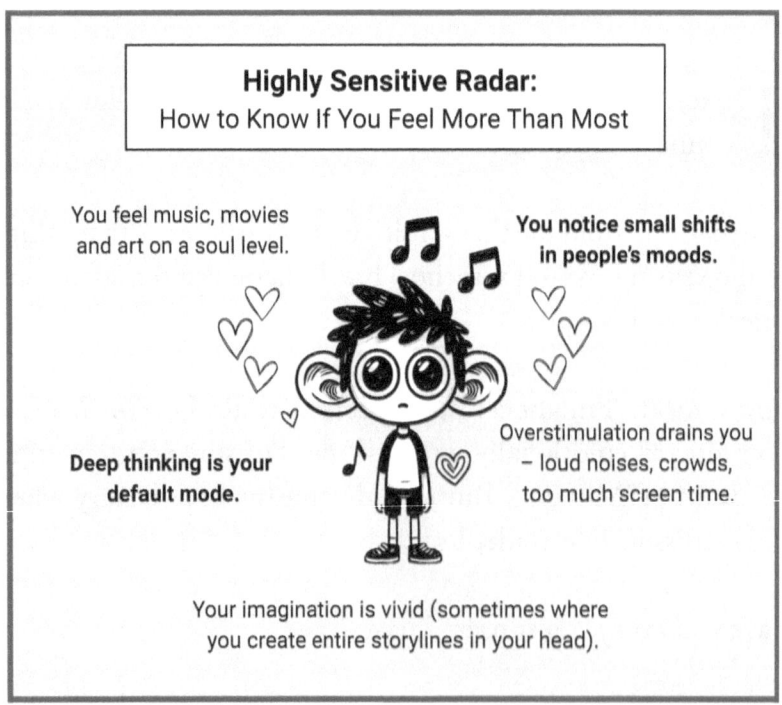

Gifts of the Sensitive Soul

For a long time, I thought sensitivity was something to hide. Society makes it seem like being sensitive means being fragile, weak, or 'too much'.

But here's the thing – the story we tell ourselves about sensitivity matters.

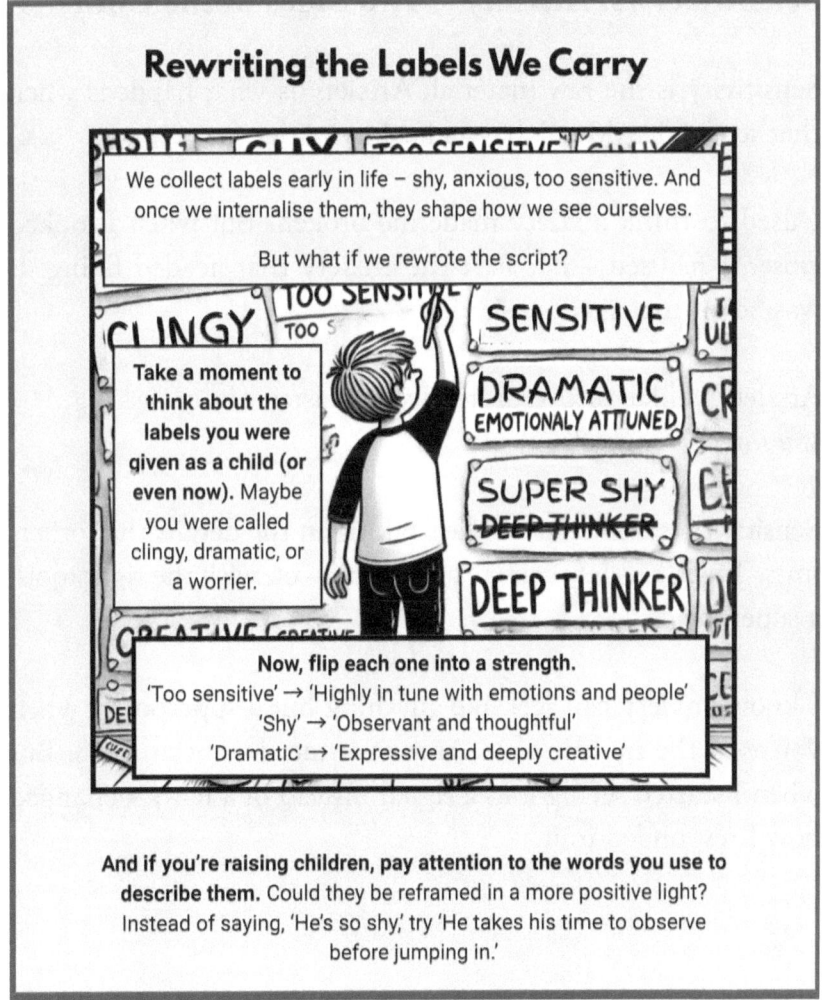

Rewriting the Labels We Carry

We collect labels early in life – shy, anxious, too sensitive. And once we internalise them, they shape how we see ourselves.

But what if we rewrote the script?

Take a moment to think about the labels you were given as a child (or even now). Maybe you were called clingy, dramatic, or a worrier.

Now, flip each one into a strength.
'Too sensitive' → 'Highly in tune with emotions and people'
'Shy' → 'Observant and thoughtful'
'Dramatic' → 'Expressive and deeply creative'

And if you're raising children, pay attention to the words you use to describe them. Could they be reframed in a more positive light? Instead of saying, 'He's so shy,' try 'He takes his time to observe before jumping in.'

The language we use – about ourselves and others – shapes how we navigate the world.

Once I stopped seeing sensitivity as a problem and started embracing it as one of my greatest strengths, everything changed.

Sensitivity vs. Anxiety – Two Sides of the Coin

Sensitivity is the raw material. Anxiety is what happens when that sensitivity doesn't have a healthy outlet.

I used to think anxiety made me broken. But when I looked closer, I realised – it wasn't the anxiety that needed fixing. It was how I managed sensitivity.

Anxiety is like an overprotective big sister, always asking, *'Are you sure about this?'*

Sensitivity is the deep thinker, taking in the details that others miss. Together, they can create a storm – or, with the right tools, a superpower.

I know anxiety can feel like anything but a superpower when you're in the middle of it. And trust me, I've been there. But when I started seeing it as a signal instead of a flaw, it changed how I responded to it.

Anxiety as a Signal, Not a Setback

Throughout this book, anxiety has shown up in different ways. As a child, it was confusion and isolation. At school, it was panic and avoidance. It turned into a cycle of running, dodging, outsmarting.

But here's the thing – I wasn't *getting* rid of anxiety. I was learning how to work *with* it.

I started recognising triggers and that changed everything. Anxiety isn't something that just 'happens'. It's my body's way of telling me something is off – whether physically, emotionally, chemically, or even spiritually. Anxiety is a messenger.

When I began listening to these messages instead of fighting them, I learnt that I could either lean in and grow (intuition) or make adjustments to bring myself back into alignment.

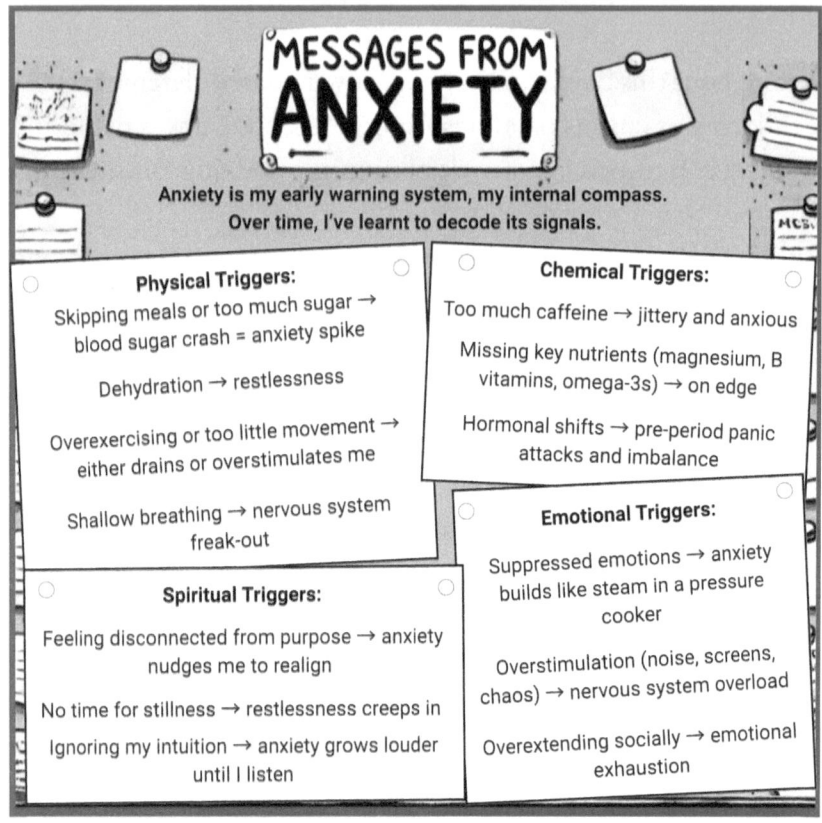

(For a more comprehensive list, check out my Free Anxiety Compass download at www.nutritionwithsammy.com.au/anxiety-compass)

For me, I've noticed that when I feel disconnected from what truly matters – whether that's my purpose, my creativity, or just quiet moments of reflection – anxiety increases. Whether you call it spirituality, intuition, or just self-awareness, I believe there's something powerful in listening to what our emotions are telling us.

I've learnt to see anxiety as a conversation rather than a battle. Instead of resisting, I ask:

What do you need?

Do you need to eat? Rest? Move? Set a boundary? Lean into something uncomfortable?

My body and mind are constantly communicating – I just have to listen.

Anxiety is my superpower. It's my early warning system, my internal compass, my personal guide. It tells me when something is off and nudges me back into alignment. It's the thing that keeps me checking in, refining, growing.

This perspective isn't about minimising how intense or debilitating anxiety can be. I know firsthand that sometimes, it feels like an unstoppable force. But in my own journey, learning to see it as a signal – rather than something broken in me – was a turning point.

Without it, I might ignore the signs. With it, I'm constantly tuning into what I need – physically, emotionally and spiritually.

Every time anxiety shows up, I have two choices… Lean in and grow or make the changes my body is asking for.

Either way, I win.

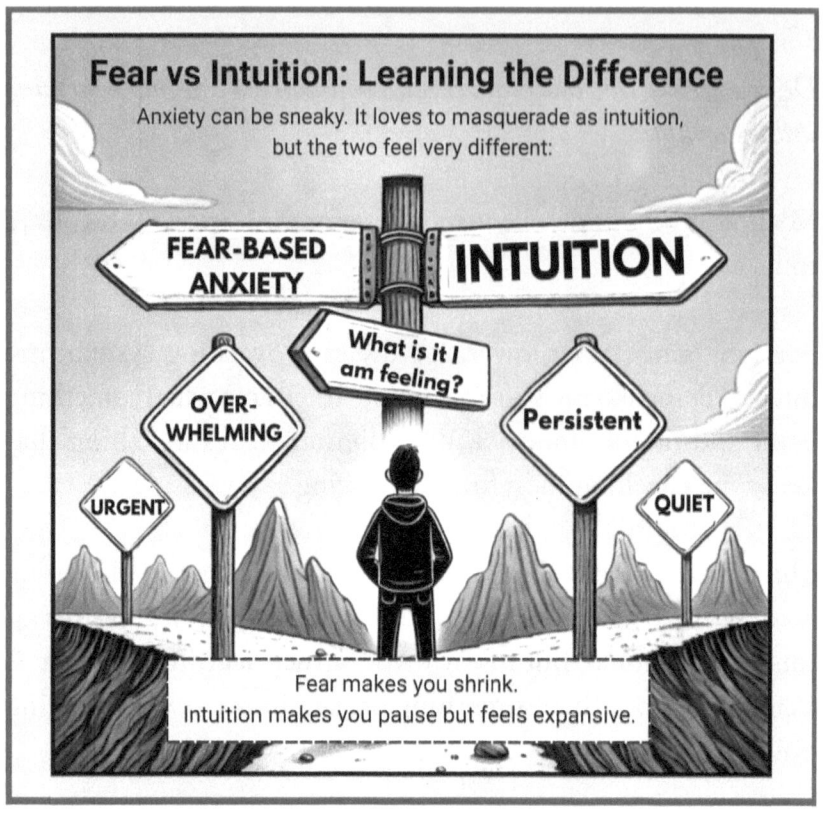

Every time I'm about to do something big – speak on a stage, publish this book – anxiety screams, *'What if you fail?'*

Meanwhile, intuition just sits there, arms crossed, calmly whispering, *'You're ready.'*

The trick is learning which one to listen to.

I won't pretend it's always easy to tell fear and intuition apart. It took me years to learn the difference and sometimes, I still get it wrong. But the more I tune in, the more I notice the patterns.

I've learnt a lot about decoding anxiety through trial and error, but I also know that everyone's experience is different. Sometimes, the best step is reaching out for support – whether that's therapy, medication, or talking to someone who truly gets it.

Building Resilience Through Anxiety

Anxiety didn't just shape me – it shaped how I parent, how I teach and how I show up in the world.

I've taken everything anxiety has taught me and turned it into my work. I help my children navigate their own challenges because I *get* it.

I teach them that avoiding discomfort doesn't make it disappear – it just delays it. Instead, I encourage them to sit with it and ask:

Why do I feel this way?

What is this feeling trying to tell me?

Our bodies often know the answer – we just don't want to listen.

Maybe anxiety needs you to *talk* to someone.

Maybe it's pushing you to do something you've been avoiding

Or finish writing this book! – which let's be real, anxiety has been breathing down my neck for years on this one.

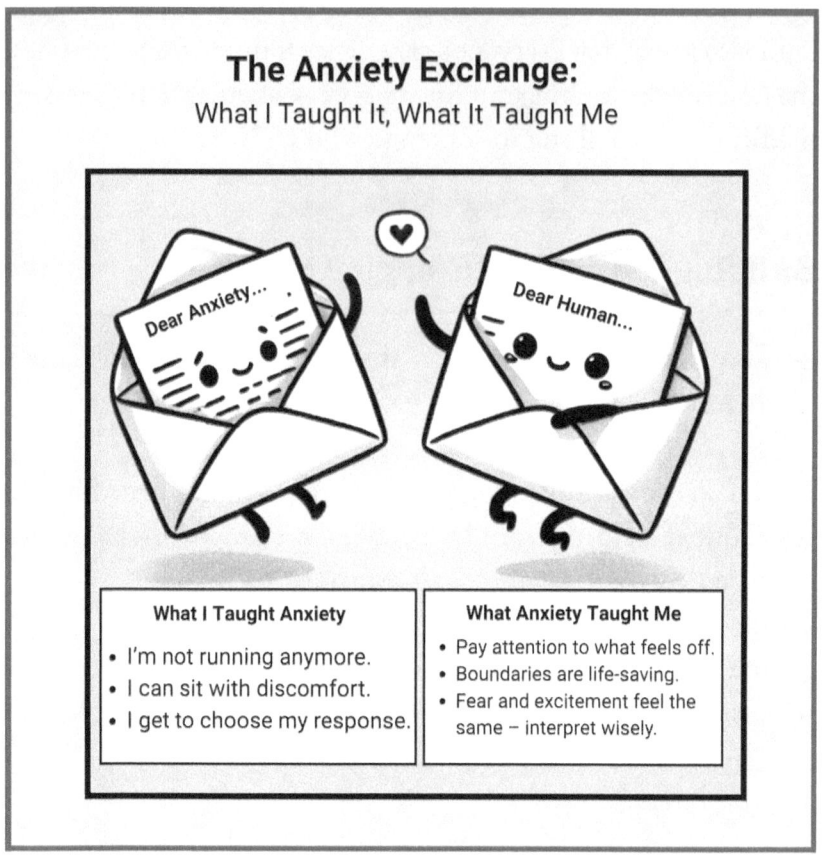

Trusting the Universe

If you're sceptical and all about the science, you might be tempted to skip this part. But I encourage you – lean into the woo.

What if life isn't just a series of random events?

What if everything – *even the hard stuff* – is happening for a reason?

Because here's the weird thing: When I started slowing down, people started showing up in my life at *exactly* the right time. Even the ones I didn't want. The ones who challenged me.

And when I stopped fighting it, I realised – every person, every struggle, every moment of anxiety is a lesson.

Anxiety still shows up for me.

I still get the odd panic attack.

I still doubt myself.

But every time anxiety shows, I ask:

What are you trying to show me this time?

I used to resist the teacher. Now? I embrace the lessons.

And some of those lessons are old – like REALLY old. So I look at anxiety and say, *'We've been through this before. Let's update the program, shall we?'*

Anxiety is no longer my enemy. It's my superpower, my compass, my (slightly overdramatic but well-meaning) guide. It reminds me that I'm alive, that I care and that I have the power to choose how I respond.

And guess what?

So do you.

The Afterfeels

If you've made it this far, congratulations! You made it through my overthinking, panic-fuelled wisdom and probably a few too many metaphors. But more importantly, you've taken the time to explore anxiety in a way that isn't just about 'managing' but understanding, growing and maybe even making friends with it.

Anxiety isn't the enemy. It may be loud, dramatic and inconvenient at times – but it's also a messenger. And once you start listening (instead of running), you realise it has some pretty useful things to say.

I hope this book has given you a new perspective, a few laughs and maybe even a little more compassion for yourself.

The journey doesn't end here.

Keep questioning, keep learning and most of all – keep choosing yourself.

And if all else fails?

Take a deep breath, chew your food properly and drink some water.

With love and a slightly calmer nervous system,
Sammy

About the Author

Samantha (Sammy) Barnett is a clinical nutritionist, speaker and writer with a knack for turning anxiety into a superpower. With a mix of humour, heart and real-life experience, she helps people understand the deep connection between food, mood and mental health.

After spending years navigating her own journey with anxiety and panic disorder, she now teaches others how to work with their nervous system instead of against it. Whether through her workshops, talks, or this very book, Sammy is on a mission to make mental well-being practical, relatable and maybe even a little fun.

When she's not deep in thought or helping others, you'll find her hanging out with her husband, kids and her highly underpaid emotional support dog, Midas.

Gratitude Roll Call

This book wouldn't exist without the incredible humans (and one very good boy) in my life.

To my husband, my kids, my mum and my sister Rebecca – you are my rocks, my reasons and my never-ending source of love (and content). Thank you for enduring my dramatic book readings just to see if I could make you laugh or at least smirk.

To my friends – especially Kassandra – thank you for hyping me up, keeping me sane and making sure I remembered to eat (a crucial role in my survival).

To my allied health crew – you've kept me grounded and helped me find my true path, even when I wandered off the tracks into the unknown.

To Midas, my furry therapist – your emotional support, judgment-free presence and ability to nap through all my existential crises did not go unnoticed.

To Stuart and the team at *Ultimate 48 Author* – my book mentors and voice of encouragement. Your insights and wisdom have made this book *so much* better. Thank you for believing in this story and in me.

To Sumiko, a gifted photographer, whose lens captured me for this book. I appreciate you and the time spent getting to know myself and my vision.

And to you, dear reader – you made it to the end, which means something in these pages spoke to you. That means everything.

With love and gratitude,
Sammy

The 'Nerd' Corner

Yehuda, R. and Lehrner, A. (2018). Intergenerational transmission of trauma effects: putative role of epigenetic mechanisms. *World Psychiatry*, 17(3), 243-257. (Page 8)

Yehuda, R., Daskalakis, N. P., Bierer, L., Bader, H., Torsten, K., Holsboer, F. and Binder, E. (2016). Holocaust Exposure Induced Intergenerational Effects on FKBP5 Methylation. *Biological Psychiatry*, 80(5), 372-380. (Page 8)

Eisenberger, N. I., Lieberman, M. D. and Williams, K. D. (2003). Does rejection hurt? An fMRI study of social exclusion. *Science*, 302(5643), 290-292. (Page 21)

Bukowski, W. M., Laursen, B. and Hoza, B. (2010). The snowball effect: Friendship moderates escalations in depressed affect among avoidant and excluded children. *Development and Psychopathology*, 22(4), 749-757. (Page 21)

Cain, Susan. *Quiet: The Power of Introverts in a World That Can't Stop Talking*. Crown Publishers, 2012. (Page 23 and 214)

Rosenthal, R. and Jacobson, L. (1968). Pygmalion in the classroom: Teacher expectation and pupils' intellectual development. *Holt, Rinehart and Winston.* (Page 23)

Poppnk, J. & Tseng, J. (2020). Brain meta-state transitions demarcate thoughts across task contexts exposing the mental noise of trait neuroticism. *Nature Communications*, 11, 1-10. (Page 28)

Aron, E. N. (1996). *The highly sensitive person: How to thrive when the world overwhelms you.* Broadway Books (Page 24)

Danese, A. and Baldwin, J. R. (2017). Hidden wounds? Inflammatory links between childhood trauma and psychopathology. *Annual Review of Psychology*, 68, 517-544. (Page 42)

Brewer, J. (2021). *Unwinding Anxiety: New Science Shows How to Break the Cycles of Worry and Fear to Heal Your Mind.* Avery. (Page 57)

Twenge, J. M., Haidt, J., Joiner, T. E. and Campbell, W. K. (2020). Underestimating digital media harm. *Nature Human Behaviour*, 4(4), 346-348. (Page 59)

Aisbett, Bev. *Living with It: A Survivor's Guide to Overcoming Panic and Anxiety.* HarperCollins, 1993. (Page 64)

Doidge, N. (2007). *The Brain That Changes Itself: Stories of Personal Triumph from the Frontiers of Brain Science.* Viking Press. (Page 68)

Brooks, A. W. (2014). Get excited: Reappraising pre-performance anxiety as excitement. *Journal of Experimental Psychology: General*, *143*(3), 1144-1158. (Page 103)

Robbins, M. (2023). *The Let Them Theory: Stop Controlling, Start Living.* HarperCollins. (Page 118)

Van der Kolk, B. (2014). *The Body Keeps the Score: Brain, Mind and Body in the Healing of Trauma.* Penguin Books. (Page 204)

Ngo, S. T., Steyn, F. J. and McCombe, P. A. (2014). Gender differences in autoimmune disease. *Frontiers in Neuroendocrinology, 35(3),* 347-369. (Page 146)

Anderson, S. C., Cryan, J. F. and Dinan, T. G. (2017). *The Psychobiotic Revolution: Mood, Food and the New Science of the Gut-Brain Connection.* National Geographic. (Page 163)

Sender, R., Fuchs, S., & Milo, R. (2016). Revised estimates for the number of human and bacterial cells in the body. *PLoS Biology,* 14(8), e1002533. (Page 163)

Strahler, J. and Stark, R. (2023). The link between rigid eating behaviors, food anxiety and mental health: A systematic review. *Frontiers in Psychology,* 14, 10490497. (Page 173)

Eger, E. (2017). *The choice: Embrace the possible.* Scribner (Page 206)

Hungry for More?

FREE: Anxiety Compass – Learn the Language of Anxiety

Anxiety doesn't show up for no reason – it has patterns, signals and triggers. The problem? Most of us weren't taught how to read them. Download my Anxiety Compass to start getting to know your body's unique language.

www.nutritionwithsammy.com.au/anxiety-compass

Book Me as a Speaker

I love sharing what I've learnt about anxiety, stress and nutrition in a way that's fun, practical and actually useful. Whether it's for workplaces, schools, or events, I offer highly engaging and fun talks that help people connect the dots between food, lifestyle and mental well-being.

Want to know more? Download my Speaker Kit:

www.nutritionwithsammy.com.au/speaker-kit

The Ultimate Anxiety Toolbox

Anxiety can feel like an unpredictable storm – so why not have a well-stocked kit? The Ultimate Anxiety Toolbox is a self-paced program designed to help you understand and support your nervous system through:

Videos: Simple, practical strategies you can use

Downloads: Tools to help you act, not just overthink

Expert Insights: A blend of nutrition, lifestyle and professional perspectives

This program takes a holistic approach to anxiety, combining evidence-based strategies to support both body and mind.

www.nutritionwithsammy.com.au/anxiety-toolbox

Notes

Anxiety: The Best TEACHER You Never Asked For

Notes

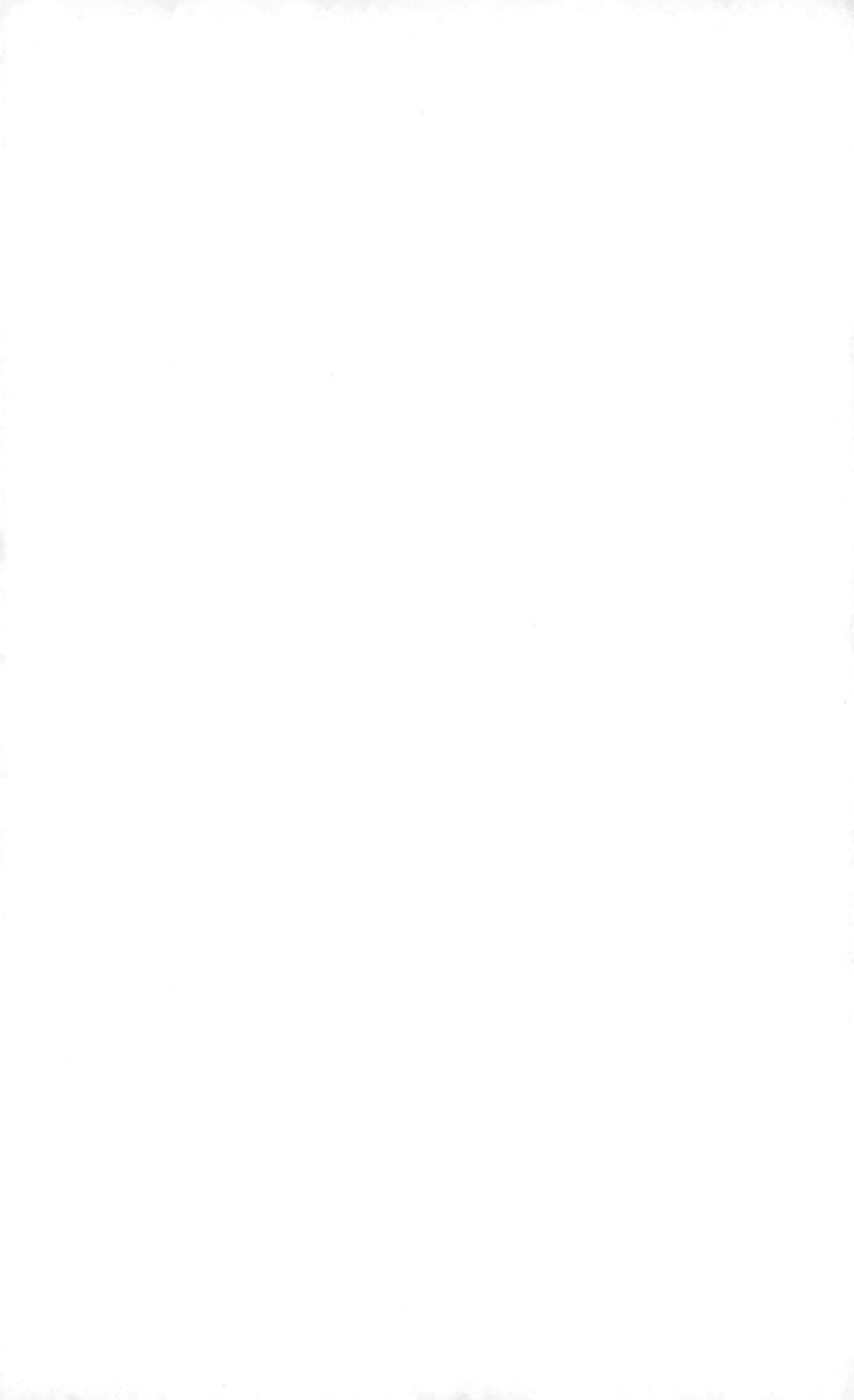

www.ingramcontent.com/pod-product-compliance
Lightning Source LLC
Chambersburg PA
CBHW020401080526
44584CB00014B/1118